DON'T MIND ME

To Audrey
Lots of Lov
Juau

D1394296

Judith
Haire

'Not a misery memoir but a story of courage
and hope.'
 Dorothy Rowe, Clinical Psychologist and
Writer

Judith Haire

Published by
Chipmunkapublishing
PO Box 6872
Brentwood
Essex CM13 1ZT
United Kingdom

http://www.chipmunkapublishing.com

Some names have been changed.

Cover Photograph by Jennifer Haire

DON'T MIND ME

For Ken

Judith Haire

About the Author

Judith Haire was born in 1955. She graduated in Political Theory and Institutions at Sheffield University (1981). She then returned to work in advertising before spending eleven years in the civil service. At 37 she suffered an acute psychotic episode which was to change her life radically. She lives by the sea with her husband Ken and their cat Smudge. Her first article was published in **Mental Health Practice** magazine in 2007. **Don't Mind Me** is her first book.

Judith Haire

Praise for *Don't Mind Me*

Over all, this is a story of hope that celebrates a survivor, and also holds lessons for practitioners

Journal of Psychiatric and Mental Health Nursing

.... leaves you with the feeling that her remarkable story will inspire others, either in similar situations to move on with their lives, or to provide a real understanding to people new to mental health.

Your   Voice   (Sheffield)

Gripping, harrowing and very brave account of what it is to experience mental illness and to overcome it.

University   Of   The Third Age

It is always heartening to read accounts of recovery. Judith's story is a valuable reminder that it is users themselves who have to shape their personal journey.

Terry Bamford, Director, SPN Social Perspectives Network

For all mental health professionals this patient insight can help us to provide a good practice for our patients and understand what they are going through aside the mental illness. This insight can also help other people whether they be sufferers of mental illness or a family or friend of a person who suffers.

Rikki Macdonald DipHE Mental Health Nurse

Inspiring and informative - this is recommended for all nursing professionals

Heather Robinson RNA

Writing in vivid and candid detail Judith Haire shares her traumatic life experiences and her journey to wholeness. Her work encourages a more compassionate approach towards understanding distressed individuals.

Dr Dan L Edmunds Ed D
International Center for Humane Psychiatry, USA

Judith's journey back to health is both thought provoking and insightful. I recommend this book to all those who are caught in the dreary slog of trying to cope with mental health problems. It catalogues this and the more dramatic entry and exit from psychosis. An easy book to read and one that shows that there is light at the end of the tunnel.

Sue Sterling Chartered Clinical Psychologist.

Judith's experiences of human rights abuses, ranging from close family members to those of the 'caring' professions, illustrates the insidious nature from which little if any recourse is found. It was simply her tenacity and determination that eventually pulled her through.

Paul P. Fletcher LLB (Hons)
Executive Director
CCHR London

Judith Haire

DON'T MIND ME

Acknowledgements

Heartfelt thanks to everyone who has given me their love and understanding. Thank you to the psychiatrists, therapists, mental health support workers, social workers and others who have helped me. Special thanks to my GP Dr Kitchener for his ongoing support. Thanks too, to my sister Jane and aunts Audrey and Shelagh for their invaluable help while I was writing this book. Thanks also to Kristina, Caroline, Gill, Denny, Jenny, Ted, Rikki, and Heather.

Judith Haire

Foreword

Don't Mind Me is the story of my dysfunctional childhood and teenage depression, my abusive first marriage and experience of rape and domestic violence, my terrifying descent into psychosis and my recovery. Writing this book has been extremely cathartic for me. It has made me stronger and helped me to see who I really am and just how far I have progressed. I wrote it to help others as well as myself and to inform mental health professionals and anyone wanting to gain an insight into mental illness.
Heartfelt thanks to Jason and Andrew and all at ***Chipmunkapublishing*** for giving me the opportunity to tell my story. To those who are suffering mental distress, keep believing in yourselves and remember there is always hope.

October 2008

Judith Haire

Introduction

The phone rang and I screamed. I was filled with terror. My heart began to pound and I started to shake. In my confused mind I had become the deaf dumb and blind boy in "*Tommy"* a film that had captivated me many years before. I moved my limbs in a stilted and robotic way. I was no longer myself. I was in a different world, the world of psychosis. I was trapped and could not find my way out.

It was 1993 and I was thirty-seven. I was entering a severe psychotic episode and this was to change my life forever. I need to take you back to my beginnings and describe how my life unfolded and how the many traumatic events which befell me made this terrifying illness almost inevitable.

Judith Haire

Chapter One: Beginnings

I was born in Kent in December 1955. My mother had met my father at teacher training college and instantly fallen for his charm. She loved him intensely but he said he would never marry her. My mother became pregnant.

She told me many years later that she had been put under great pressure to have sex and on that particular occasion she knew it was a fertile time of the month for her and neither she nor my father had any contraceptives with them. My father ignored her worries and continued to put pressure on her, saying he would kill himself if she did not have sex with him there and then. She found the pressure too much to resist.

Because my father was studying for exams she hid her pregnancy selflessly for several months and when she eventually told him all hell let loose. His mother insisted it was a deliberate act to trap him into marriage. My father broke down and demanded I was aborted.

My mother felt an overwhelming sense of duty and responsibility and decided there was no option for her but to marry my father. The wedding took place at the end of July 1955. My mother had just turned twenty and my father was twenty three.

Once my mother went to live with my father in his parents' house she saw a totally different side to him. His fury at having to marry her manifested itself in a regime of punishment – moody silences, cruelty and snide remarks. Once I was born, life became even worse for my mother. My father's abuse of my mother was always unpredictable and would usually occur in the winter months, with sudden unprovoked bouts of rage. My father acted as though I did not exist. He ignored my presence totally. We all shared a bedroom. My mother said those first four years were hell.

My paternal grandmother Maud was, I think, torn in her loyalties and turned a blind eye to her son's awful behaviour towards my mother, while she was pregnant with me and after I was born. My mother was frightened of my father and vividly recalls her unwilling compliance to have sex when he was in a rage.

My parents decided that if I was born with dark hair they would name me Juliet and if I was born with fair hair, Judith. I was born with golden red hair actually. My second name is Frances. When I was very young my father would tease me that I was baptised "Cess." My surname was Pool and I felt hurt by this comment.

My mother was dreadfully unhappy cooped up in one room and living in her in-laws' house. She would often stand looking out of the window, crying and wishing she could be somewhere different.

From what she has said in later years, she certainly never regretted giving birth to me. It was the marriage to my father that she bitterly regretted as it brought her so much pain and unhappiness.

She tried her best to leave my father when I was four months old, taking me in my pram, her belongings hidden inside, but did not get very far before she was consumed with guilt about deserting him and made her way back home. She had planned to travel to Dorset to live with her mother and father. To the rest of the world my father was charming and nice but to my mother he was not.

Chapter Two: Growing Up

For the first three years of my life I shared the room with my parents, sleeping in a chair that folded down into a single bed. Unconsciously I must have absorbed much hostility, noise and conflict.

My treat was to go downstairs to the dining room and sit next to my granddad, Jack, and eat a saucer-full of boiled brussel sprouts sprinkled with salt and pepper. I still love sprouts, especially when they're cold.

Jack was a lovely grandfather. He had lied about his age in order to enlist for the army during World War 1. He never spoke to me about his experiences in the War but I guessed he was traumatised by them and I think this was why he was always suspicious and a little paranoid about life in general. When I was older I remember him noting the registration numbers of cars parked outside his home and chalking them on the brickwork in the lean-to. As a young child I remember him working long hours in a factory and that he always supported Charlton Athletic. There was a piano in the house and Granddad used to play his banjo.

Almost from day one I had continued to absorb the undercurrents of discord between my parents. My father never forgave my mother for falling pregnant and continued to punish her throughout the twenty three years of their marriage.

My parents' marriage was dysfunctional as my father related to my mother as his mother not his wife. He expected her to do everything for him, just as a parent would do, and would be prone to tantrums if he did not get his own way, almost like a toddler. Much later on, my father's psychiatrist said to her, "Do you really want to be his mother?""

My father was also involved in a love affair with a female work colleague and one day he brought this woman to the family home for a meal – it was as if he was introducing a girlfriend to his mother. The woman stayed overnight in my bedroom while I was not there. My father had put chocolates and flowers in the room and during the night he left the marital bed and went into the spare bedroom while his children slept in the next room. He then calmly returned to the bed he shared with my mother. My mother suspected there could have been encounters with other women too.

After my father was born his mother was very ill for several months with a depressive illness and my father was looked after for three months by a friend. I am certain this early separation from his mother is at the root of his own emotional difficulties. He didn't start to talk properly until he was four and until then called everything "gravy".

I am told he was very clingy and would often get into his mother's bed in the morning after he had finished his paper round. This continued until he was about fourteen. My father's parents had not married for love either. My grandfather Jack said he had married Maud, when thirty, because he was "hungry".

I adored my paternal grandmother, Maud. I called her Nanny. She was a depressive herself and often looked quite unkempt and hopeless but I still loved her dearly. She was one of thirteen children and had been brought up in grinding poverty. Her parents had turned to the local Catholic Church and to the nuns for help in bringing the children up and, as a mark of gratitude, six of the children were converted to Catholicism.

Nanny had a strong Catholic faith and prayed with rosary beads and kept containers of Holy Water. She went to Church as much as she could and would sometimes take me along with her. I found this strangely comforting.

Maud insisted I was baptised. My father had gone abroad on a school trip but my mother took me to Dorset and I was baptised there.

My grandfather Jack's pet name for me was "Ju Ju" and he was fiercely protective of me. One day I was playing under the table. I was about two and stood up suddenly, hitting my head on the corner of the table. I cried out. "That will never happen again," said Jack and went straight outside, returning with a saw. He sawed off each corner of the table and sanded the wood to a smooth finish.

Maud was one of my carers, looking after me sometimes while my parents were at work. She took great interest in my daily development which compensated for the fact that my father ignored my presence. He complained constantly about my crying. My mother had to keep me quiet. I have since wondered if this suppression of my crying was in part responsible for my chronic tonsillitis as a toddler which resulted in a tonsillectomy when I was eight. I can still remember the acute post-operative pain and the many times I vomited blood.

My father was insanely jealous of me when I was a baby and resented any time my mother spent with me. He once slapped my mother across the face when she was breastfeeding me.

I have vivid memories of being very young. I remember being in my pram at the end of a long garden belonging to a friend and calling for my mother but she was looking the other way and did not hear my cries. I felt very anxious. I was ten months old. At three I remember getting lost outside my aunt's London flat. I had strayed from the back garden and could not find my way back again.

And I was accident prone as a child. At two I fell in the bathroom and had an horrendous nose bleed. I was taken for an x-ray which was very painful as I had to lie face down. I was under two when I had to have surgery to correct a "trigger" thumb. Maud had been the only person to notice that I always kept my left hand closed in a fist, as I could not straighten my thumb.

I had a fascination for Maud's garden and in particular the huge peach tree and the plants called Red Hot Poker. Somehow I confused these with the real poker in the fire place and one day pulled the poker out from the embers and was saved from scarring by Maud promptly applying a poultice of bicarbonate of soda to my palm.

Another time I fell and cut my forehead just above my eye and still have the scar, in my eyebrow. One day I had been given a balloon and the string was blown from my hand while I was out shopping with Maud and my mother. Spontaneously I ran out into the traffic to try and retrieve it. This put Maud and my mother into a state of shock and made my father very angry.

At only twenty months old I was sent to a childminder as Maud's eyesight was deteriorating and she went on to have cataract surgery. At only two years of age I transferred to a nursery school. I can still remember how much I hated going to this school. The staff were very strict and unfriendly. One morning I showed my displeasure by kicking and smashing the windscreen of the motor bike side-car I was taken to school in. I still remember the humiliation of being punished severely at nursery school but I was too young to verbalise what had happened to me.

When I was three and a half we moved away from Maud and Jack and into our own house. I was bereft. Though I still saw them when they visited us, it was a very different life without them and a great upheaval for me.

We had holidays with Maud and Jack and we went to holiday camps and also to Ramsgate where we stayed in a boarding house and I took my first faltering steps on roller skates.

I was three when we went on holiday to Dorset and I still recall sitting in the paved back garden of my maternal grandparents' house. As a small child I loved walking and could manage as much as six miles in a day.

I will always remember family gatherings at Gran's house. The bathroom ceiling was white and my aunt Shelagh had decorated it herself with red handprints. Shelagh and her other sister Audrey were very good tap dancers and they would tap dance on the table in the dining room while singing "Tip Toe Through The Tulips".

One Christmas, when I was about five, we were all gathered round the dinner table when my mother's younger brother said something my father deemed offensive. My father told him off. This in turn offended my grandfather who said he was head of the table and of the family and it was up to him to tell his son off, not my father. There was an unpleasant atmosphere after that and when we left to return to Kent, my grandfather would not shake hands with my father. From then on we never spent Christmas in their home again.

I continued to have accidents, falling head first down the stairs and being saved from crashing through the glass door panel by my inflatable yogi bear, a present from Maud. It had saved me but I was sad it was no longer inflatable after my fall. Another time while in Gran's house, I ran down the hallway and fell onto some empty milk bottles, gashing my shin quite badly.

Growing up was an emotionally painful time for me and I often had trouble sleeping at night. My mind would be crowded with horrible thoughts and memories and sometimes I would tell my mother about them. She said I must imagine a big screen that I could pull down inside my mind and cover all these thoughts with, and then paint them all out using black paint. I used to try this technique and it worked. She said it had worked for her too when she was a child so I didn't feel quite so alone when I knew this.

I have often wondered if my father had really wanted me to be a boy. My mother has since said how glad she was she didn't give birth to any boys for she is convinced my father would have bullied them even more badly than he bullied us. My father made me building blocks from lengths of wood and spent time telling me about the stock market and making me miniature share certificates. Of course I was too young to understand what he was telling me and would become upset when he took the certificates back from me saying he had sold the shares.

At five I became very ill with measles and a fever and experienced my first hallucinations, seeing little furry squirrel-like animals, climbing in and out of holes in the bedroom curtains. I also had a frightening nightmare at the same age, where the whole of the house was ablaze and I could actually smell the smoke. I have since wondered if that fire was symbolic and a sign of suppressed anger.

I clearly remember the night in January 1962 when my sister Jane was born, at home. I heard her first cry and was able to see her in her cot, yawning, when she was only a few minutes old. I was excited to have a baby sister but of course it was another great upheaval for me. I am sure now that because my mother's second pregnancy was calmer and happier, Jane was born a less anxious baby than I was. I was told she cried a lot less.

Later that year we all moved again, to the coast. My father's brother had already moved there and my father had a tendency to follow his older brother's lead, having already followed him into teaching as a career.

It did not strike me as strange, until I was older that my mother never saw our new house until the day we moved into it. My father and his brother looked at various properties and my father only took me with him to see the new house, shortly before we moved.

When I saw the house which was to be our new home, my heart sank. It looked dingy with sombre black paintwork on the outside and inside was dark chocolate brown paintwork and depressing dark red and cream flock wallpaper. The weeds in the back garden were waist high. The inside of the house smelled rank and there were carpet bugs on the floor.

It was August when we moved and Jane was seven months old. She slept in her pram throughout the move. This time I was even more sad as we were so far away from Maud and Jack and it was a happy day for me a year or so later when they moved to live in a bungalow near us. My security was restored somewhat, though life was still dreadful at home.

Growing up continued to be tough. I was an anxious child, prone to nail biting, sore throats and worrying needlessly. I had a fantasy that really I had been adopted and my real parents were lovely and were waiting for me somewhere else. I was convinced I was going to die when I was nine as I had heard of a nine year old child who had died from burns and I thought something terrible would happen to me too. I was highly relieved when I woke up, alive, on my ninth birthday. I had the usual childhood mishaps, plenty of falls and at five I had visited Buckingham Palace, tried to get a closer look at the changing of the guards and got my head stuck firmly between the railings.

I experienced my father as angry and moody and he took out his feelings on my mother, shouting and raving at her. Sometimes he hit us and we all lived in an atmosphere of fear. I often came home from school to find my mother in tears. She would try to cover up and say she had a cold but I knew why she was crying. I heard her crying in the night sometimes too. We never went without food but often went without fun and laughter and my father's sulks and rages were the norm. My mother suffered from constant tension headaches and bad throats.

One day we were expecting my aunt and uncle to arrive. Whenever visitors came my father would be especially tense before they arrived, very nice to them while they were here and then as soon as they left our house, he would revert to his usual stern and unapproachable self. On this particular day my sister Jane and my mother were having some sort of argument and my father shouted at Jane to shut up. He then heard her talking to my mother, but this was about something else and in his rage he grabbed Jane by the top of her hair and shook her by her hair and in the process she banged her head on the door post. My mother stood watching this. My father, still in a rage, carried Jane upstairs and threw her on to the bed. She was five. My mother recalls that my father often picked me up as well as Jane and threw us both on to the sofa when in a rage. I wondered if other families were like this and was aghast when I visited my school friends' houses and saw, in fact, how happy their lives were.

My father had spent long hours during his own childhood sitting on the step outside the pub, waiting for his parents to finish their drinks and take him and his brother home. He remembers family parties and how his eyes would water with the thick cigarette smoke wafting round the room. He decided not to follow in his parents' footsteps and has always been very critical of those who like to drink alcohol. Consequently he only allowed my mother to have two drinks at a time, and only on special occasions. The sherry was kept locked in the sideboard cupboard.

There was a family meal when I was in my teens and my aunt and uncle came to eat with us. My father had bought one large bottle of wine for everyone and it did not last long. Seeing a little left in the bottle I shared it round while he was out of the room and he was absolutely furious with me and sent me a letter berating me for interfering and using up the wine and warning me of the dangers of drink.

My father's mantra was, and still is, "Life Isn't Easy". His glass was always half empty.

We were not allowed to have friends to play with us or stay with us. It seemed to me my father hated his job as a teacher. He said he was fed up with seeing children all day long so when he got home he wanted peace and quiet. My mother's demeanour would change as soon as he walked back into the house. She would appear frightened and meek. My father would walk straight into the kitchen and close the door. We would hear his raised voice. If we wanted anything we had to knock on the kitchen door. And then we would be sent away. There were many times when I wished my mother would stand up for us against our father but she was too frightened. Her fear of him was so great it seemed to immobilise her. She stayed with him far too long and we all suffered the consequences.

My father's temper was easily provoked. He always seemed angry. He kept a punch bag hanging up in the garage and he often went there to vent his rage. We were relieved when he did this as we were spared his vile temper. My father has since said he only used the punch bag for exercise.

When I was eight I went to piano lessons and would practise my scales on the piano at home. I struggled with the theory of music but was good at playing the piano, as Jack had been. The piano I practised on was chopped up for firewood by my father and I thought this was bizarre. He later told me it had been chopped up to make more room.

I heard that an aunt said of me when I was ten "I wonder if she will survive". My father ruled the family by fear. His eyes shone cruelly as he shouted at us. His foul moods filled every corner of the house. When I was ill with a cold he put Vick on my tongue. I still recall the discomfort.

I felt I never had any privacy growing up. My parents' bedroom adjoined the bathroom and my father would listen from the bedroom when I was using the bathroom and count how many times I was pulling toilet paper from the roll and then tell me I had used too much. We had little money. We had few holidays. There was little or no fun or laughter, trust or compassion so instead I threw myself into my school work and excelled.

At the age of ten I decided I would like to learn to dance. My mother had little or no spare money but she generously paid for my lessons. She was able to earn some money by doing some supply teaching.

I went to dancing school three times each week to learn Stage, Tap and Ballet. I have several certificates for the exams I passed and also a Bronze Medal for Tap. When fifteen and revising for O Levels my anxiety levels were high and I stopped dancing.

My one solace was our cat Sambo. He was only six weeks when we got him and had clearly been taken away from his mother too early as he used to suck and nuzzle at anything woollen. He became very ill shortly after we got him and one night my mother was convinced he would not make it to the next day but he rallied and grew into a handsome black creature. He was a good friend and I was heartbroken when eventually he had to be put to sleep.

My outings with my friends were another treat for me. Up until I was around ten I was allowed to go out on my bicycle and to spend time with two friends as long as I went to their homes. I loved cycling and passed the Cycling Proficiency Test with 96%. Later I used to cycle to and from school in the summer months. But even so my father tried to undermine my attempts to cycle and said I was "as nervous as a kitten."

My new   primary head teacher had decided I could miss a year so I was one of the youngest in the class and when she later told my parents I was to sit the eleven plus a year early I was very unhappy as I still struggled with Maths and really wanted to repeat the final year to give myself a better chance. But did my wishes matter? I sat the eleven plus and tried my best to fail it. Even so I passed   and fear turned to dread when I won a place at the local Grammar School. Maud was visibly proud of me and my father simply snapped that children would give their right arm to be in my place - something which I doubted.

The school uniform was very costly and the list of equipment was endless. We even had to wear a pair of "indoor" shoes. My mother did not have the money to buy another pair of shoes so she dyed a red pair of shoes brown and I wore those around the school instead.

I hated the Grammar school from the moment I set foot in it. It was like going back in time. I found the atmosphere in the school oppressive and archaic and grew tired of being told we were the "cream". Impossibly high standards were set, for me, at least. I had so much homework. I did not know where to start and I used to sit at my father's desk in my parents' bedroom poring over my books while my father played his LP *The Sound of Music* very loudly downstairs. He played the LP over and over all evening. I hated every song. I cannot bear to listen to the songs nowadays and feel sick if I hear them and cannot watch the film.

In the summer of 1967, at the end of my first year at Grammar school, my mother gave birth to another baby, my youngest sister. I remember being astounded that she was having another baby. My father told her she had not consulted him about the pregnancy and refused to speak to her for a week when she broke the news. That was what he was like. Of course my mother's sisters were furious, I later learned, for now it would be more difficult for her to leave the marriage and she would have to wait for the new baby to grow up.

Our neighbours' children all had German measles so it was decided to leave my baby sister in the hospital until all risk of her catching the illness had passed. This separation really distressed my mother and she used to spend as much time as she could at the hospital. I had to go on a school trip to Hampton Court so was not at home the day my new sister was brought home. I helped all I could to look after her which was a welcome diversion from the strict regime at school and at home.

The birth of my youngest sister turned my life upside down. A new baby in the house meant upheaval in an already chaotic life and my sister's cries would resonate through the house and make concentrating on my homework even harder. My mother worked very hard in the home and was even more exhausted by the demands of a new baby, and my father hardly welcomed my youngest sister's presence. The extra work I had to do in the house took   its toll on me and sometimes I struggled to cope with this life change which had been thrust upon us all so unexpectedly.

As I developed,   the time came for me to have my first bra and I still recall the humiliation I felt when my father demanded that I lift up my clothes so that he could see it. This made me feel very vulnerable.

Chapter Three: More on My Teenage Years

My unhappiness continued and when I was thirteen Maud was taken into hospital. She was very ill with thyroid carcinoma and was not expected to live. My last and enduring memory of her is when I stood at the foot of her hospital bed, with my youngest sister in my arms, and she smiled at both of us. She was wearing an oxygen mask but I saw the smile in her eyes. I never saw her again. She died a couple of days later and I was inconsolable .She was only sixty-five.

I was completely distraught when Jack said no grandchildren were to go to the funeral and being forced to go to school that day broke my heart. It was the saddest day of my life. I was not allowed to say goodbye to Maud. I cried and cried. I still feel let down.

I was allowed to visit the grave later that day and still visit the grave where she has since been joined by Jack. I think of them often. Just recently for no reason at all, the framed photo of their headstone fell off my bookshelf.

Maud's death was something I could not recover from. More tears flowed. I started to hear voices in my head. I would hear a deep booming male voice in the mornings; I could never make sense of what he said and did not know until later in life that the voices were my own thoughts. I had constant sore throats. I continued to cry, I neglected myself, I wasn't sleeping well and was struggling even more with school work.

Without my knowledge or agreement, my mother went to the family doctor who referred me to the Child Guidance Clinic. My father had started taking me to school in the van to make sure I went, and one morning he made a detour and we arrived at the Clinic. My father waited outside while my mother took me in to see the doctor, a psychiatrist in a white coat.

He gave me some aptitude tests and said there was no reason why I could not do my school work. He then asked me many probing questions about my home life, suggesting there was trouble at home and between my parents. I vigorously denied this and staunchly defended both parents. Such was my mother's fear of my father she denied there was any trouble either. I am still extremely angry about this experience. The psychiatrist could get no further so he prescribed *Diazepam* to quell my anxiety. I was already taking *Mogadon* to make me sleep. Problem sorted, or so the psychiatrist thought. In those days there were no bereavement counsellors. I was medicated and labelled a psychiatric case.

As a child I felt I never deserved anything good in life. I felt that everything in the world was there for other people and not for me. I felt that clothes in the shops were for others and not for me. When I listened to the radio it felt as if people were speaking to everyone in the world except me .I stayed on medication for the next two to three years. I know things are different these days and this would never happen to someone so young now. But it happened to me.

At fifteen I left school with seven good O Levels, which was a miracle considering I was living in such a stressful environment and I had taken the exams a year early. My father had been to the headmistress and asked that I be taken out of Maths and Geography classes as he said I wasn't coping with nine subjects. I know very well I would have coped superbly had things not been so dysfunctional at home.

My father then refused to let me go back to the sixth form, deciding for me that I would not cope. He would say of me, "she's in a state". Or if I got upset or tearful he would say I was spoiling his day, He would say in later years, "forget the past". It is not always so easy.

I went to college to study beauty therapy and hairdressing with Art and English but left after six weeks. I felt I didn't fit in. My depression worsened. Everything was grey and hopeless and there was nothing to look forward to. My father was having a severe nervous breakdown, the first of two. During these breakdowns he was at home for weeks and weeks and grew his hair and a beard. He cried constantly. He would hide behind the hedge to avoid seeing passers-by. The atmosphere in the house was indescribable. Jane was around eight years old at this time and says it was like bedlam. My father was crying, I was crying, and my father would be totally unmoved by my distress. Jane remembers me being beside myself and my father shouting at me. There were some really bad scenes at this time.

Eventually at sixteen, I was well enough to start a clerical job, which I loved, in an estate agents, and my boss wanted me to study for the qualification of FSVA (Associate or Fellow of the Royal Society of Valuers and Auctioneers). I missed my school friends who had stayed on in the sixth form and envied them as they were allowed out to the folk club, the pub and parties and I was not. I was very upset about this. I was already fearful of boys; my mother had made sure of that. She told me to be careful of boys and their "desires" and if I saw a boy walking towards me I absolutely froze inside. Of course she was terrified I would become pregnant like she did.

I went to evening classes and learned silver work, metal work and basketry and I learned to drive and passed my driving test first time, but otherwise led a very limited and lonely life, going to work, going home for lunch, and living an awful life with my family. I still loved my music and was given a small Spanish guitar and slowly taught myself the chords and to play a few songs.

Things had deteriorated so badly at home the only chance I had of saving my sanity was to give up the job I loved and move away to London. The psychiatrist wanted me to move away from the family. I was eighteen.

Recently I was able to go through my medical records and found the letters this psychiatrist sent to my then GP. He described me as "inadequate". I wish he could see me now. I wonder if he realised all those years ago that one day I might read what he had written. The move to London was arranged for me and I was to live with my aunt Shelagh.

Chapter Four: London

I had my own room in my aunt's house and I soon made it very untidy. I still feel ill at ease if things are too neat. Clutter makes me feel more secure.

My aunt and uncle did their best to make me feel welcome but I always felt in the way and as if I should not have been there.

I was like a fish out of water living and working in London. My aunt said I seemed frightened of everything. I was young and naive and everyone I worked with seemed so sophisticated. When I overheard a colleague describing me as "gauche", I felt awful. I was constantly anxious and would often worry that I could smell gas escaping in the street.

I had already taught myself to touch-type and I went to classes after work to learn shorthand and passed two exams.

After ten months living in my aunt's house I was very pleased when my good friend Maggie moved to London to work and we decided to look for a flat together. This took three weeks and during this time Maggie stayed in my aunt's house too.

We found a room to share in a flat which took up the top two floors of a terraced mansion just off the Fulham Road. There were five women in the flat and it was chaotic. There were few rules and it soon became a pig sty. There were maggots in the kitchen and mice in the bedroom. It all became too much. My family visited one hot summer day and my father was appalled at the state of the wiring, which was bare and dangerous, and he made it safe.

I went home most weekends and my father continued to undermine me and blame me for all the discord. Jane said it wasn't all my fault. One weekend I was unwell and did not go back to work in London on the Monday so phoned my employers to tell them. I was very upset at having to miss work. My father sneered at me as I made the call and said he couldn't understand what the fuss was about, saying 'You're only a typist '. That comment hurt. I was secretary to two account executives and one account director.

In 1975 I went with Maggie and three other friends for a week's holiday in Cornwall. I was still awkward around men and never knew what to say. Some of my friends commented that I didn't talk naturally and what I said sounded rehearsed. This was a blow to my already fragile confidence and I did not know how to improve things.

When we got back to London Maggie and I went out with some girlfriends and I met Ben and started my first relationship. It ended while still embryonic. I really took heed of my mother's warnings. He wanted me to have sex with him and I felt shocked that he should ask me. I really did not have a clue about men and was heartbroken when he finished with me.

Maggie found us a room to share in another flat in Notting Hill Gate and she moved in a few weeks before me. This flat was lovely; a surprisingly airy semi-basement and there were four of us sharing. Everything was more controlled and civilised and I was much happier there. One day I returned to the flat after work and found the front door open. We had been burgled. Nothing had been taken but the entire flat had been turned upside down and cartons of milk had been poured all over our beds. This really frightened me and added to my general sense of insecurity.

After two years of flat sharing and working in the advertising agency, I began to acknowledge how angry and resentful I was that my father had prevented me from returning to school. So I gave up my secretarial job and returned home to live and go to college for a year.

Chapter Five: Home Again

I was forced to start the course some six weeks into the first term as I had a painful throat virus. One day I was in so much pain I couldn't get up and stayed in bed until late morning when my father walked into the bedroom and forced me to get up. As soon as I was well I travelled by train to college each day,   studying A levels in English Language and Literature and A and S Level in History.

It was not easy living at home again and trying to study. My sister Jane was studying for her O levels and we encouraged each other to keep going. My father once walked into the room   late at night when I was reading and just closed all my books .On the morning of one of the exams my father was not speaking to any of us again and had gone off in the car. I got into the exam room feeling very anxious and sat for several minutes before forcing myself to start writing. I finished the exam early and when I told my father this,   he said "well you won't have done very well then".

My parents went out that night which was a rarity.   I had brought home a bottle of gin. Discouraged by my father's thoughtless remark and by life in general I drank too much of the gin and passed out cold.   Jane refilled some of the bottle with water to try to hide this from my parents but when they got home I was still out of it and had to be given hot black coffee. I was throwing up and rambling. My father panicked and phoned the local hospital for advice and also phoned my gran. The next day he was still fuming with me. My then boyfriend arrived to spend the weekend with us and when I said we were going out for a drink my father said that had I been a boy he would have knocked me out for saying this.

Despite the problems I passed with grades A, B and Merit. I had a place at Southampton University but got cold feet and returned to my old job. During my A levels my boyfriend had dumped me for an older and more experienced woman and I had the pain and rejection of that to cope with too. I stayed with my aunt and uncle again for a few weeks before moving into a flat.

I was sharing with strangers and I hated it so much. There was no communal sitting room and the other two women were cold and distant and complained about cooking smells so I had to eat cold food. I found the evenings very lonely. I would meet up with Maggie one evening a week which lifted my spirits but otherwise I would sit in my room watching television and go to bed early.

I met up with Bridget a good friend from college, and she was enjoying life at University in London and she said to me, "you're like a satellite where you are. Why don't you give up your job and re-apply to University?" I didn't need to think about this for long and applied through the Clearing System.

I rang round the Universities myself and spoke to the Professor of History at Sheffield University .He said with such good grades at A level I would be offered a place there and then. By this time I had given up the flat I detested so much and was staying at a friend's.

I worked out my notice and went home for a week. With my encouragement and my sister's encouragement, my mother had found a flat to rent. Each day she cycled there to take things she had smuggled out of the house. She did not want to leave the family home until she was sure I was safe in Sheffield. She came with me to the station and saw me off. That was a wrench. When I rang that evening to say I was safely in Sheffield, my father answered the phone and asked if I was phoning from Southampton. That was the extent of his interest.

Chapter Six: Sheffield

I moved into the Hall of Residence and got involved in Intro Week and registered for my first year subjects – Politics, History and German.

The following Friday my mother told my father she and my two younger sisters were going to stay with her sister for the weekend. He went to work and as soon as he had gone, her friend came with a small van and moved all their belongings into the flat.

That night my father rang my aunt and asked to speak to my mother. My aunt said my mother and sisters were very tired and had gone to bed. On the Monday night my father's world was turned upside down when my mother rang him and said she was not returning. My gran had walked with her to the phone box and supported her while she made the call. My father broke down. He moved in with his brother. Three months later he was living with his new partner. They are still together. My mother continues to live alone.

When I had arrived in Sheffield I didn't know what to expect. It was cold and wet and rained every day for the first fortnight. While I settled into University life I heard from home quite often and it all sounded very traumatic. My youngest sister was eleven and became a tug of love child. I was far away from my dysfunctional family and the freedom was liberating.

Most of the other students were northerners and southerners were few and far between.

Judith Haire

The University buildings were twenty minutes walk from my Hall. I really enjoyed exploring the city.   I couldn't take in how huge Sheffield was. There were so many parks and so many amenities. The pace of life was slow   after the rush and tear of London and the city was cleaner. At twenty-two I soon found other mature students to be friends with and I was enjoying life for the first time ever.

I went to my mother's flat for Christmas. On Boxing Day my father and his brother came to see us. My father collapsed in hysterics and I had to walk through the snow to the phone box and call out the doctor. My father said he wanted oblivion. The doctor gave him medication and my uncle took my father home. My father was still sobbing.

I went back to Sheffield for the start of my second term but soon felt unwell. I was taken into the student clinic with flu like symptoms. I was bleeding too. I had no energy and was very depressed and could hardly get out of bed. I was told to get up but couldn't. I had a stabbing pain in my right shoulder and realised it could be linked to problems in my fallopian tube or ovary.   The doctor dismissed my concerns and said I must have been sleeping in a draught.

Some of my fellow students came to see me. The doctors said I had depression. My friend Andrew went to the nurse and said he thought there was something really wrong with me and that I wasn't normally like this but usually bright and cheerful.   Another friend said the room smelled of illness. Anyway no one listened, my bleeding was dismissed and I was sent back to the Hall. I became worse and the warden called the doctor out to see me. I was doubled up in pain and he was unable to examine me so he rang his colleague, a gynaecologist at the Jessops Hospital for Women. I took a taxi to the hospital and was too ill to pay the driver – I did so later on. I could hardly make it up the stairs to see the gynaecologist.

The gynaecologist tried to examine me but I was in so much pain it was impossible. She said I could be pregnant. She asked me when I had last eaten and immediately ordered an emergency D & C (dilation and curettage) and an emergency laparoscopy. An instrument called a laparoscope would be passed into my abdomen to investigate. I had a throbbing pain in my right groin as I waited to go to the operating theatre. After the emergency operations the gynaecologist said my cervix was blue and I had a very high white blood cell count indicating infection. No pregnancy was found but she could not even see my right ovary; it was completely obscured by what appeared to be an abscess but was actually the swollen fallopian tube. Afterwards I had a small puncture wound in my side where she had drawn off some of the contents of the tube for culturing.

Nothing grew on the culture and I was given antibiotic injections every few hours and then had to take antibiotics for a month. The gynaecologist told me the abscess had been developing for a very long time. I was in a lot of pain after the operation but the gynaecologist was pleased to see me up and washing my hair on the second morning. She said that was definitely a sign I was getting better though I was still very weak and had no energy. My recovery was slow but sustained.

While in hospital I heard that my grandfather Jack had died. He was eighty one and had suffered a second stroke. I had to miss his funeral, which saddened me. I was actually snowed in; and conditions were treacherous. The lady in the next bed had to have a termination very late in her pregnancy and her husband had walked eight miles through the snow and ice to see her.

I failed one of my first year exams as I had fallen behind with my studies and revision. The gynaecologist had written a letter to the University saying I would have to take things easy while recovering and as I only failed the History by one mark I was upset that the department had not given me a pass. I had to re-sit the History exam and I went home to my mother's house and revised. At that time my gran and granddad lived in the next road and I went and stayed with them for a week. I had total peace and quiet to revise and my gran cooked all my meals.

I now rented a room in a shared student house so I had to travel up to Sheffield before the start of term to take the re-sit and was on my own in the house for two days and nights which added to my anxiety about the exam.

I passed the re-sit and decided to change faculties and study Politics. I had passed the German exam and received a certificate.

I was still emotionally upset about my time in hospital. The gynaecologist had said I'd also been suffering from depression which had made it all the harder for the doctors to spot the gynaecological symptoms. My friend who was studying law put it to me that the doctors at the student health centre had been negligent in my care and had left things for too long before taking any action and I could take out a case against them. My fallopian tube could have ruptured and this could have been fatal. I still did not have the strength to do this but I was upset to find that, in any case, all my medical notes had gone missing.

All went well as I started my second year and I passed the exam in Statistics, which boosted my confidence after all my earlier difficulties with maths. In my spare time I sometimes helped out with the student newspaper which gave me a taste of working life again.

I had to go back to London to be available as a witness in a court case after a taxi I was in the year before was hit by a passing car. I was not called to appear in court. So I was able to meet Jane and we also met my aunt. I was able to catch up with what had been happening at home .

Back in Sheffield I met Don, a mature student. and started going out with him, staying some of the time at his flat in Rotherham. He was very secretive. He refused to give me his phone number. One day at my house he said he was going out to buy milk and did not return. He had gone home.

One of my house-mates told me he already had a girlfriend. Don had been seen leaving the girlfriend's flat one morning. By now I had managed to find his phone number on a student notice board and phoned him. A woman answered. I had already found a nightdress under the pillow and lipstick marks on a cup and he said they were both his sister's. One morning I had arrived unannounced at his flat and he wouldn't let me in – I had wondered why I stayed over so infrequently. If he stayed at my house it would be for an afternoon, rarely overnight. That was it. I felt humiliated and used but it was difficult to shake this man off.

He would phone me and hang up when I answered. He got into the back garden in the early hours one day and threw stones at my window. I found the whole episode distressing and became depressed again. It wasn't only this relationship, it was everything that had happened at home, catching up with me and I started to fall behind with work again.

I was referred to a psychiatrist who said I had been flattened by my father and should never have been referred to her. She prescribed me medication and I went to see my lecturer to discuss what I should do.

He said I had a choice. I could take a year off or carry on. He said for the sake of my psyche he would recommend I carried on. I took his advice and did, knowing my results would suffer and they did, I got a Third Class Bachelor of Arts Honours degree in Political Theory and Institutions where I had been expected to achieve an Upper Second Class. But I had the degree, that's what counted, and against all odds.

In July 1981 I heard the news that Maggie had given birth to a baby girl. I went to London to visit her and meet Eleanor. I am truly proud to be Ellie's godmother and she is now a successful graduate and businesswoman herself.

Chapter Seven: Troubled Times and Back to Sheffield

After my degree I left Sheffield to live with my mother and youngest sister. I plunged into depression. I was medicated again but this time was very concerned about the side effects and burned all my tablets. I had stopped the medication too suddenly and was very sensitive to light for a few days and wore dark glasses. I was otherwise lucky to be unscathed.

Things did not work out.. I was always in conflict with my mother and did not get on with my youngest sister. I gave up my part time job as Assistant Organiser with Age Concern and headed back to Sheffield. I stayed at a friend's for a few days and another friend told me of a room to rent which I took. I had applied for various jobs before I left my mother's and had been offered a fortnight's work in a Sheffield advertising agency. I was told I was like a breath of fresh air! The fortnight was extended to a month and then the job was permanent.

The shared house was great. There were four other women. Julie lived in the front room with her cat, Tiger. She was a post woman and was always home when I got back from work. I would have a cup of tea with her and we would chat. In the evenings she studied Psychology A level and would use me as her subject for experiments. I would score so highly the whole correlation of results would have to be changed. She went on to take a degree in Art Therapy following her Fine

Arts Degree and I am still in touch with her. She now lives in Ireland.

I continued to work as receptionist and secretary in the Sheffield advertising agency and assumed more and more responsibility. I was given the responsibility of moving us all to modern purpose built offices in the city centre. I wanted to use my degree, to use my skills and asked my boss to promote me to production assistant, to which he agreed. He then reneged on his promise so I handed in my notice.

I did not have another job .Unemployment was rife in Sheffield in l983. I sat a number of interviews but got nowhere and became dispirited. What kept me going was the fact that my new housemate Geoff was also out of work. He was an ex-miner and very anti-establishment and very cynical but he had a wonderful sense of humour like mine and we got on well. He died tragically at 32 but I am still friends with his former girlfriend.

In the evening paper I saw an advertisement for a free government course to help me find a job. I applied for a place and started the course and was interviewed on closed circuit television and trained in interview techniques. This course made all the difference and at the next interview I was selected as temporary marketing assistant with the Manpower Services Commission in Sheffield. I'd become a civil servant.

I loved my job in the Marketing and Information Branch. Many staff had re-located from London which was good. I travelled to London a couple of times to set up exhibitions and went to marketing meetings in Manchester. My job involved organising the publication of training manuals, arranging exhibitions and advertising.. Really my life could not have been better. Each night my housemates and I took turns to cook. Life was good. After six months I applied for the permanent post along with two hundred others. I was shortlisted and got the job.

I continued to have a wonderful life but it was all to change. I had to go to London for a week's training and chose to stay at my uncle's flat rather than in a hotel. There I met my future husband.

DON'T MIND ME

Chapter Eight: Clinton

On 6 March 1984 I met an ex-boss after a day on the course and got back to my uncle's flat   quite late in the evening. I was going straight to bed but my uncle had two male friends there and I was introduced to them. One of them, Clinton was to become my husband. Clinton was Trinidadian. He was very attentive to me that evening. Later in the week I heard he wanted to see me again and he called round to the flat again later in the week. At this time I was oblivious to the extent of his feelings for me.

I had to return to Sheffield on the Sunday. My uncle and Clinton came to see me off. As I waved goodbye from the train, I felt confused and tearful .Clinton rang me very late that evening and again the next morning and we spoke often in the week. I knew he was married and I had his phone number and there were times when he was unable to speak to me and would call me back. He asked me to go back to London to see him at the weekend.   Something pulled at me to go but there was an undercurrent of doubt which I refused to acknowledge.

I had already started neglecting my many friends in Sheffield,   such was his power over me. I even cancelled a week's holiday in Spain. I had paid for the holiday and was going with a girlfriend but I cancelled and   reimbursed my friend.

I started going to London every Friday night, after work. It cost me a fortune but I didn't worry about that; I felt a compulsion to go and see Clinton. One Friday night I arrived in London to be met by my uncle saying he would take my bags back to his flat while I went by underground to East London to meet Clinton at his house. His wife was on a night-shift. She was a nurse. Clinton was looking after his son. My uncle warned me not to oversleep and with that he was gone.

I made my way to East London thinking all the while, this was dangerous, and I shouldn't be doing it. I arrived at the house and went into the living room. Suddenly the front door burst open and in rushed a small thin woman. Her face was lined with worry. She gave me a hostile look and then she and Clinton fought furiously.

I looked on in horror. Clinton picked up a heavy glass ashtray and repeatedly smashed it into his wife's face, cutting her badly. She had grabbed a kitchen knife and brandished it at him. They screamed at each other and wrestled. I stood frozen to the spot.

Clinton shouted at me to go upstairs and get his clothes. I went up the stairs and found the main bedroom, and grabbed one pair of trousers before becoming so petrified I ran downstairs where he shouted at me to go outside.

I know I should have left the scene and gone straight back to Sheffield. Clinton's wife had climbed over the back wall and gone to her neighbour's. Clinton joined me in the street and we made our way back to my uncle's flat and told him what had happened. It was the next morning that the full horror of what had happened hit me. I knew there would be implications. Clinton got a court summons. His wife had taken out an exclusion order, banning him from going within five miles of her and their son. She had also written to the Immigration Authorities and said she was disowning him.

I felt overburdened with responsibility and doubt. I hardly knew Clinton and had now seen how violent he was. Yet I felt I had to help him; I felt responsible for the fight and the ensuing trouble between him and his wife.

Clinton was now homeless. He came back to Sheffield and stayed with me. My landlord did not like him but just about tolerated him. Deportation proceedings had started and we had to attend many meetings. We went to the Joint Council for the Welfare of Immigrants, for support and advice, and were assigned a solicitor. Meanwhile Clinton was being petitioned for divorce by his wife on many grounds, including his adultery with me.

It was now April 1984 and Clinton made my life very difficult because he resented me going to work while he was left on his own. And yet he relied on me financially. He would threaten me; if I did not leave the office at 5pm he said he would go back to London. I was too scared of him to go against his wishes and complied all the time. I found it hard to concentrate on my work knowing he was waiting outside or wandering round the City, spending my hard-earned money. My work suffered. Money was short because I had to pay for a whole new wardrobe of clothes for him and also pay for his cigarette and alcohol habit.

It was not long before Clinton raped me while we were in the attic room. My housemates were downstairs, I screamed out loudly but they did not hear me. I bitterly regret not going to the police right away and reporting it. I will never understand why I didn't. My housemates tried their best to dissuade me when I said I was leaving Sheffield and moving to London to live with him. But "love" was blind and I couldn't see what I was doing wrong.

I have since wondered if I was set on a course of self-destruction. I had countless opportunities to leave the relationship but I felt trapped and had an overwhelming compulsion to stay.

Acting on impulse, I gave up the job and house and transferred to a government department in London, leaving most of my belongings in Sheffield. As soon as we arrived in London I started my new job and was unwell on the first day. I did not return to work for six weeks.

For six months we stayed with my uncle at his flat and the rape and violence continued. One morning, after a particularly savage beating, I was passing blood and took myself to hospital. I underwent several investigations and it was found I had cystitis which was no doubt exacerbated by the stress I was living under.

One night we had been out with friends and were walking back to a friend's flat for coffee and had stopped to buy some fried chicken. Clinton was a very possessive and jealous man and became angry because I was walking ahead talking to our friend Alan. He threw his food over a hedge and sulked.

Once in Alan's flat Clinton became uncontrollably angry and threw me across the room. I landed awkwardly, breaking some fingernails and ripping my tights. He then lunged at Alan. We got back to my uncle's flat in the early hours as we had missed the last train home, and when he saw the state of me he was furious and said he wanted no more to do with Clinton.

We moved into our own flat in Blackheath in November 1984. Without my uncle things were very different and I felt as though I no longer had any protection from Clinton and his violent nature. Clinton raped me again and one morning I woke up to find he had inserted a deodorant roll- on inside me and this was painful to remove.

I struggled to afford to buy furnishings for the flat. Clinton was very moody and if I said I didn't like something he had chosen, he would storm out of the shop. I quickly learned to swallow my feelings and let him choose everything. It reminded me of living at home with my father. I still had to pay for Clinton's cigarettes and alcohol. And I also had to give him money to buy materials for his costume designing. My designs were as good as his, any day and I often had to go shopping for materials and help him with the project.

There was never any money left for me to buy food at work so I had to work all day when very hungry. Usually I had some cream crackers for lunch while Clinton would tuck in to any leftovers from the meal the night before. He drank heavily and frequently, often starting at 9 a.m. I had to walk a good part of the way to my job in central

London, to save on fares, and part of the way home again too.

Each morning when I left the flat for work I let out a sigh of relief. I had a few hours' respite from the torment while I was at work, and then I had to return to it in the evening. I was constantly miserable and depressed. Occasionally I would catch sight of myself in a shop window and be shocked at how drawn and defeated I looked.

Clinton and I both belonged to the Greenwich Arts Council and through this committee we met Carl, another artist. He was gay and despite this Clinton was very jealous of my friendship with Carl who had told a friend that had he not been gay he would have married me.

One night, we had been for a meal at his flat and out for a drink and later that evening back at the flat Carl and Clinton started to row. I tried to intervene and calm things down but to no avail. Clinton lost his temper completely and started to smash his fist into Carl's face; blood pumped from his nose and spattered the walls and my beige raincoat. I screamed at Clinton to stop and he did eventually but Carl was in a bad way for many days afterwards and I felt terrible.

Clinton also turned upon my uncle on several occasions and beat him up too, once breaking his ribs. In later years I was to find out that he had beaten my uncle "many, many times". It is possible that these beatings are responsible for the subdural haematoma now threatening my uncle's life.

Clinton and I were staying with my mother and youngest sister for the weekend when Clinton crept into the room where my sister was sleeping and tried to molest her. She woke screaming. I refused to believe it had happened at the time, but later I had to admit it had and felt truly awful. Clinton then exposed himself to my sister Jane on the landing in her house and she told me some time later. Again I was horrified. He also tried to molest two of my friends. He borrowed money from my father which he never repaid.

Clinton designed costumes for the Notting Hill Carnival and expected me to help him make the costumes every evening after work. We always worked until midnight at the earliest and soon fatigue overtook me and I found it very difficult to get up early to go into work. I struggled with my work as I was always so tired and worried.

Being in a mixed-race relationship was never easy and I encountered much prejudice from his friends. I was called a "middle-class white" and learned to keep quiet in social situations.

Foolishly I married Clinton in May I985. He had booked the wedding in April before his decree absolute had arrived and I had forced him to cancel the booking. There was no money for a wedding reception and we were only accompanied by two witnesses. There wasn't enough money to buy wedding rings but I bought my own eternity ring though I stopped wearing it soon after we married.   On our wedding night I said to him: 'I don't fancy you'. I married Clinton mainly out of a false sense of duty and fear.

Marriage to Clinton sealed my fate; the rape and violence continued. I would often go to work bruised and sore. His alcoholism worsened. One night when drunk he flew into a rage, grabbed me by the hair, threw a drink in my face and then proceeded to smash all the pictures on the wall with a hammer. Then he demanded I lie down on the floor with my legs open all the while brandishing the hammer. I lay there terrified but he didn't do me any more harm that time.

Clinton often invited friends round and they would stay late, drinking and making a noise, playing loud music. I would go to bed and try to sleep, knowing I had to get up early in the morning for work. He ignored my pleas to stop these late nights. Early in the morning, especially if it was a Saturday or Sunday he would get up at seven and hoover the flat, forcing me to get up too. He refused to go to the bathroom in the night and used a bucket which he kept by his side of the bed and expected me to empty in the morning.

Things would be difficult when his son came to stay over. At six years old, he did not understand why his father had left him and his mother, and was understandably very angry and had to have counselling. He often wet the bed. I found him difficult to control.

Throughout 1985 and 1986 the violence, alcoholism and mounting debt continued. We were behind with the rent on the flat and were lucky to keep it. Somehow, against all odds again, I was promoted at work and so was relieved to have more money coming in each month.

Looking back, my marriage was as dysfunctional as my family life and upbringing had been. I had married a bully and a sexual pervert who was verbally abusive too. Eventually I was mentally destroyed. My confidence had been eroded, and being hit and concussed took away my sense of self-worth. What added insult to injury was the day Clinton urinated in my mouth and laughed afterwards. He did not work and if he did the odd project now and again, he would spend all the money on alcohol. I was exhausting myself trying to make ends meet.

Clinton had taken control of me from the very beginning. He would choose the clothes I wore and buy me clothing with my money. I did not like the choices he made for me but being frightened of his violent temper made me comply. He stopped me wearing make up and nail varnish and dictated how my hair was styled. He threatened that if ever I was unfaithful he would injure me so badly internally that I would be unable to have sex again. And yet he was unfaithful to me.

In 1986 I went to Sheffield without Clinton to collect the belongings I had left when I had suddenly upped and left in 1984. My friends had kindly looked after everything for me. I took the opportunity to tell my friend Heather exactly what I was enduring and she was very supportive.

During the same year I started to tell my family what I was going through. I would have my mail sent to me at work to stop my husband opening personal letters. My manager at work had an idea things were not right with me. I had taken a lot of time off work through illness and to sort out my problems and he told me to my face I was an "unfortunate character". My welfare officer, on the other hand, was very kind and counselled me every week in the lunch hour.

My mother would send me money each week so that on Friday after work I could catch a train and go to stay with her for the weekend. It was my sanctuary to stay with my family. When things got really bad I would go home overnight in the week too.

I went to see a solicitor for advice and phoned a women's refuge. I was at an all-time low, and one Saturday morning I made myself admit I could do no more. This was a turning point for me. I realised things were not my fault, would get no better and I couldn't change Clinton. It was 5th December 1987. I packed a few things in a weekend bag and left. My husband assumed I was going to my mother's as usual and as I hesitated at the front door I asked him not to harm my things. He just snapped at me that if I was going to go, I must go. I left behind nearly all my treasured possessions; I just had to escape.

I cried all the way to the station and all the way to the coast on the train. I cried every day for a month. I would walk three miles to the seafront and back, crying all the while. Clinton used every manipulative trick in the book to persuade me to go back to him; he said he had bad chest pains, he said he kept hearing footsteps outside and thought it was me. Once he had accepted that I had left for good, he then refused to let me go to the flat and get my belongings. Even though I enlisted the help of a solicitor eventually I had to give up trying to get back my things. He told everyone we knew I had gone to live in the country with my uncle. Eventually, some years later, I did retrieve some things after he had abandoned the flat. The council had packed everything up and put it all in their store and I was able to collect some things but he took many of my favourite possessions and my birth certificate, degree certificate, marriage certificate and jewellery. My dear gran had given me a lovely gold pendant watch and a lovely silver and aventurine ring; he took both of these.

I have often been asked why I stayed with my first husband. I feel I had grown up with an enormous sense of responsibility and I felt I had to see things through. It was as if I had been conditioned in my early years to love too much. I felt to blame for the situation I found myself in. I felt I couldn't leave him; what would happen to him if I did? I felt controlled and manipulated and felt so unworthy it was almost as if I deserved everything that was being thrown at me. It was almost as if I was repeating the pattern set for me by my mother. I had unwittingly married a version of my father.

Even before we married, Clinton had admitted to having sex with another woman quite early on in our relationship and after I left him, I discovered he had been sleeping with people of both sexes during our relationship. Shocked, I went to the hospital to ask for an HIV test. I had the blood test and was asked to return for the result in a fortnight.

That fortnight seemed like a lifetime. My sister Jane came with me to get the result. I went into the doctor's office, highly nervous and terrified at the thought that the result might be positive. Jane says she was very anxious herself and could hear her heart beating loudly and wondered why I was so long talking to the doctor. She could only assume it was bad news. But then I emerged, smiling. The test had been negative. I still remember the relief I felt.

Chapter Nine: Toby

Reviewing my life after I had left Clinton, I had to decide whether to go bankrupt or carry on. I decided to carry on. I thought time would heal. How wrong could I be. After only four weeks' sick leave, I went back to London to work and commuted two hours each way. Soon afterwards I was able to transfer to a job near where I was living. I was made manager of a scheme offering grants to small firms and also gave advice on a range of export and other services for businesses.

I was not at my best. I felt an underlying anxiety which gnawed away at me and I went to see an Osteopath as I had severe back and hip pain. After the first treatment I cried uncontrollably for a week, hyperventilated, was very anxious and had neck pain. When I saw the Osteopath again I told her about the break up of my marriage and she said she wished I had told her that initially as she would have given me a much gentler treatment. She has since said that my reaction to the treatment was not usual and was in keeping with my having suffered the abuse that I went on to tell her all about.

I became involved in another relationship; it was a classic case of "on the rebound". Toby had two failed marriages behind him and was averse to working and a heavy drinker. He was not violent though. Again my family had reservations about my choice of partner.

During 1988 I had decided to seek psychotherapy to help me get over my problems.

I was assessed and allocated a trainee therapist called Mary.

I was not too confident driving at the time. Though I had passed my test first time as a teenager I had only just started driving again, for my new job, and so Toby would drive me the twenty miles to my therapy appointment and wait outside in the waiting room. Mary was very disapproving of this arrangement and explained that therapy was something I had to undertake alone and so I plucked up the courage to drive there and back alone. As Toby liked to go to the pub most evenings Mary became concerned that I was drinking too much alcohol and suggested it could be interfering with the therapy.

Against my wishes Mary organised an alcohol assessment for me at a local hospital and I went along for my appointment. The male nurse greeted me with "what's your problem?" I replied that I did not have a problem and that it had been my therapist who had arranged the meeting.

I had to tell the nurse exactly how much alcohol I drank and how often. He told me that the man he had seen before me was drinking two bottles of whisky a day and that really I was not drinking that much in comparison. He said that drinking altered one's moods artificially. But he advised me to give up alcohol and finish my therapy.

I did not get any support from Toby who took the view that no one could tell me to stop drinking and if I wanted to have a drink, then I should. I used to go for a drink so that I would be in the same frame of mind as Toby.

I went to therapy with Mary a few more times. We did dream work and I painted some wonderful pictures of my dreams in the sessions as well as many beautiful pictures at home. But my therapy was being compromised by my alcohol consumption and Mary said I could only continue for a further month. I was very sad at the last session and took away my collection of art. I tried to carry on without any therapy and continued to find life very difficult indeed.

In the summer of 1991 my grandfather Frank died and we were all very sad. He had written his first book at the age of eighty and was ninety when he died. Toby and I went to his funeral and his ashes were scattered at sea.

But by October 1991 my life was so full of problems that I picked up the phone and rang the alcohol unit and said I needed to give up drinking so that I could resume my therapy.

My first appointment was with a wonderful male therapist called Paul. I saw him every week for almost two years. He was my lifeline. I told him my meetings with him on Friday afternoons "punctuated" my week. I still keep in touch with him.

At our first meeting he told me there were two ways to give up drinking. One was to stop drinking immediately. Another was to limit my intake to two drinks in a session for the next six weeks and then stop, for good. I decided on the first option and found it quite easy. This surprised me. I had thought I had a dependency on alcohol but the reality was different and this made me see my relationship with Toby in a new light.

Paul recommended that I read two books on co-dependency and I was shocked to find out the truth about my relationship with Toby and it made me realise my relationship with Clinton had also been co-dependent.

At this point in my relationship with Toby there was no longer any intimacy and the relationship was heading nowhere. I was angry and resentful at his drinking and continued refusal to hold down a job. Our money was short; I had bought the house from Jane and was falling behind with the mortgage repayments. I was being threatened with repossession. The relationship did not feel "right".

During the relationship with Toby I often suffered terrifying nightmares and often woke up in the night shouting. The anxiety continued. The anger and resentment grew and grew as I struggled to pay all the bills while Toby continued to be out of work and drink in the pub all day and most evenings, if he was not playing snooker.

I was suffering from headaches and when I told Paul, he said "You have to find a voice. No one can hear your headaches." During those two years the anxiety gradually built up in my body. I suffered from depression too. I realise now that depression is anger turned inwards. Paul also said to me, "You have to learn to live with your depression, rather than in it."

I had hoped my emotional wounds would heal but the anxiety only increased and the emotional pain was gradually getting the better of me and manifesting itself in the form of physical aches and pains and in 1992 I had to take five months off work with severe back pain and sciatica. I found myself immobilised by pain and had to have two weeks' bed rest before the physiotherapist could even start to work on the problem. I became even more depressed. The trauma I had suffered during my marriage stayed with me and inside me and I still could not bear to look at any television coverage of the London Carnival – so painful were the memories it evoked.

Chapter Ten: Alone – Descent into Psychosis

In July 1992 Toby and I split up for good. We had parted for the first time in January l990 but had got back together in the April. I knew I had made a serious mistake in allowing Toby to move back in with me. I felt responsible for him and tried to carry on as best I could.

By October l992 I didn't really feel quite right but tried to ignore how I was feeling. I travelled to Sheffield by coach and stayed with three sets of friends, a couple of days with each. One of the friends was Sheila, the girlfriend of my late housemate, Geoff and she had a dog which was later destroyed for viciously biting her. The dog had a kind of epilepsy I believe. Anyway on my first evening at her house the dog bit me on the arm. I was in agony. I had always had a fear of dogs as, when I was a toddler, a dog had jumped up at me in my pushchair and frightened me badly. I still have a scar from the bite. Luckily I'd had a tetanus booster shortly before going to Sheffield.

I went to stay overnight with Julie and Jim and we all went to the cemetery to look at Geoff's grave and leave some roses there. I wasn't entirely sure of the grave's whereabouts and was wandering around feeling a bit helpless when I called out, "Geoff where are you?" and within seconds I was standing at his grave. It was a weird feeling. After a few days I returned home by coach. One couple wanted to come and visit me the following month. Whereas normally I would have welcomed their visit and set a date, this time I tried to put them off, saying I was worried about the weather. These particular friends had no experience of depression and did not really understand. But I couldn't have coped with these friends coming to stay with me. I felt too vulnerable by this stage.

I continued to work full time. I gave a presentation to a large audience of business people, I organised exhibitions and seminars, I drove all over Kent visiting companies. I tried to carry on as normally as I could. I went on two week long residential courses in the south east. I drove to Essex to see some friends. But deep inside the pain and anger raged, gradually consuming my soul.

It was during 1992 that I was reading 'Beyond Fear' by Dorothy Rowe in which a man was telling her that he was worried he had touched a child but was sure he had not, and as I read these words a hot, searing pain shot up through my lower body. It felt as if I was being sliced in two. I never found an explanation for this phenomenon. I told Paul my therapist and he listened intently.

On 5th December l992 it was exactly five years since I had left Clinton and I was able to file for divorce. I drove to the county court myself and handed in the papers and felt overwhelmed by relief. I regretted that I had not filed for divorce in l989 when we had been separated for two years but at that time I had not been strong enough mentally or physically. Now in l992 I did not need Clinton's consent.

At the beginning of l993 my anxiety really began to escalate. The future of my job was in doubt and since I was settled by the sea I did not relish commuting to London again. Hindsight is a wonderful thing. Looking back I can see I was already heading for the episode that would throw me so dizzily off balance and make me feel as if I had left this planet.

If only I hadn't tried to keep my feelings hidden after the break up of my first marriage and also after the break up of the subsequent relationship, perhaps things could have been different. I had made the mistake of trying to be strong, of not talking about my experiences, of hoping the pain would go away, the flashbacks would stop and life would return to normal.

My sister Jane was expecting her first baby in May l993. I had been upset when I first heard of her pregnancy. At the time I was having gynaecological problems myself, problems which had started when I was fourteen. I was supposed to have had an exploratory operation at that age but I'd been terrified and the operation had been cancelled. These problems were still being investigated and I found my sister's pregnancy difficult to cope with. I tried to suppress my negative feelings and went swimming each week as normal with Jane, and her ever-growing bump, and tried to look cheerful and stay positive.

Shortly before Jane gave birth, Toby rang sounding distressed. I asked if he wanted money but he said no, he had taken an overdose of hundreds of *paracetamol* tablets the night before.

He arrived at my house, ghostly white, and I took him in my car to hospital and he was sent for a stomach-pump and admitted to a ward.

Jane and I went to see him the next day and he looked far healthier, sitting up in bed, reading a paper. I did not visit again and heard he had been admitted to the psychiatric unit. He phoned me, trying to pressure me into visiting him but I made it clear we had split up. He later discharged himself. I catch sight of him occasionally but have no contact with him.

The day Jane went into labour, I was at a meeting in Chatham and I called into the Maternity Unit on the way home, hoping to see her and give her some encouragement. I saw her husband, Tim who said it wasn't possible to see Jane at that moment but I left my mobile phone with him so he could call people with the news later on. At nine-thirty that evening Tim rang to tell me Jane had given birth to a healthy boy. Despite all my reservations, I felt exhilarated and couldn't wait to see the baby the next day and to see Jane. Looking at photographs of me holding her baby when he was a day old still makes me feel strange. In the photos I was smiling broadly and looking perfectly healthy and yet only six weeks later I was hospitalised.

At the beginning of July 1993 I had to drive to Peterborough for a two day residential training course. Normally I would not be anxious about this but as I set off from my house at five in the morning tears were already streaming down my face. I managed to get through the first day of the course, but the next morning I had to get a grip of myself and tell myself I would be all right. I had to say out loud "Judith, you are in Peterborough and you will be okay!". I drove back home and returned to work to discover that the following week I would have to drive to Leeds for another course. I was very scared about this. I made tentative arrangements but my heart was not in it.

My good friend Caroline told me later that one of the most shocking things about my illness was that she had had hardly any inkling that I was ill at all.

She said I was always so capable in my professional role. I never really talked to Caroline about my personal circumstances –our conversations were mostly about what we were doing work-wise.

Caroline recalls having lunch with me and my telling her that I was seeking a divorce from my ex-husband. She realised how nervous I was that he might come to find me. She also noticed I had lost a lot of weight but at the time I was not consciously dieting.

The "inkling" came to Caroline because apparently, I had said to her rather casually that I was worrying about waking up in the middle of the night with an important thought and then being unable to remember it in the morning. Caroline suggested I took a pen and a pad of post-it notes to bed with me so that I could note anything important. Hearing this now makes me realise I was more ill than I thought at this stage, because saying this was so out of character for me.

The events I had lived through in the period 1984 to 1987 were to catch up with me very soon. I had booked a week's leave from work and on the Friday evening as I locked away my working files in the cabinet in my office, I knew I wouldn't be coming back to this job.   That realisation surprised me yet I knew it must mean something

During my week's leave, Caroline came and visited me one evening. She still remembers the sinking feeling in her stomach as she walked into the basement room and saw written-on post-it notes covering the walls. This was only a day or two after her suggestion and she knew this was a disproportionate reaction from me and things weren't right.

On this occasion I seemed slightly strained to Caroline but certainly not unbalanced in any other way and she said later how she struggled to understand what could be going on. She had the impression I was now virtually living in my basement.

I started to feel even more on edge. I ate little, I hardly slept for the week, I stayed dressed as I was so full of energy. I was alone in my house, and started to experience   visual and auditory hallucinations. The fear grew and grew and I was imagining all kinds of horrors were going to befall me.   I opened the back door to be physically knocked back by a rushing crimson and gold tornado hurtling towards me; such was the power of my imagination. I imagined all kinds of sinister meanings in the newspaper headlines; I imagined the editorial was all about me. I imagined there was a nuclear war going on around me, I imagined my house would explode the next time I opened the front door.

One of my hallucinations was about a Fabergé Egg fashioned in gold and filigree and black and at one point this opened into two halves and I had the feeling I was at the mid-point in something. During this hallucination I was on the phone to a national newspaper and they were laughing at me because I referred to it as the Daily Jellyfart and then I suddenly started to sing "Don't Cry for Me Argentina" while pivoting from foot to foot. I was on a high; the energy rush was amazing – yet the extreme terror I experienced was suffocating.

Some of the hallucinations were in brilliant colour, and music played all over my body. Red and green waves of colour shimmered all around the room. My behaviour and beliefs became bizarre. I had regressed to a child-like state. Yet I would lapse into fluent French or German.

The carpets and furniture would take on different textures and meanings to me; suddenly everything would appear "frosted" with huge three dimensional icy structures on them and they would come alive and threaten to swallow me up. The fear I felt was indescribable.

At the end of the week I began to imagine my chimney was on fire. I actually phoned the fire brigade who came to check on it and said it was fine. A friend phoned me and soon realised how ill I was and phoned my mother who came to see me and stayed overnight with me. The next morning she called my GP who came to see me. I was lying on the bed. I had washed my hair twice that morning and had taken all my clothes of the wardrobe as I was unable to decide what to wear. I had piled all the clothes on the bed. I knew who the doctor was   and realised he was trying to help me by suggesting I went to the psychiatric unit. I was so overwhelmed with terror that I refused, saying I didn't want to end up like a zombie. I will always remember how he shrugged his shoulders helplessly and said that he would have to leave me then, lying in a mess.

Some time afterwards,   I said sorry for refusing to co-operate and he said he had understood.

Chapter Eleven: Hospital

My mother stayed all day. By late afternoon I had become worse. Another GP came to see me and arranged my admission to the psychiatric unit. My youngest sister drove the three of us the twenty miles to hospital. I curled up on the back seat. I was admitted to the Unit the night of Saturday 17th July 1993. The hospital was a red brick Victorian building set in spacious grounds and as we parked I was still curled up, oblivious to what was happening to me.

We went inside the building which was very dark and dingy and were led into a nurse's office where my mother spoke at length and I sat saying nothing to begin with. But I did not know what the date was or who was Prime Minister. I thought there were bombs in my back garden and that I was part of a plot to assassinate the Queen. Eventually I was taken to a dormitory and got on to the bed and curled myself into the foetal position, closed my eyes and tried to shut everything out. I didn't look at my mother and sister again and they left. Though I didn't really understand what was going on, I felt abandoned.

Years later I asked to see all my medical records and was astounded to read the report made at the time of my admission to the psychiatric unit. There in spidery handwriting was the comment "had been binge drinking" and "two bottles of spirits a day". To this day I have no idea where this idea had come from. I would certainly not have said anything like this, it simply was not true. I had not drunk any alcohol since October l991.

I awoke the next morning, somewhere else, asleep on the floor of a large room. I had taken my bedclothes with me and I had no clue as to where I was. I was hallucinating, that I was back at the Grammar School and this was the assembly hall.

I was taken to the dining hall where there were other patients. My parents came to see me that morning though I have no memory of their visit. My father wanted to take me home but I was too confused to understand. My mother realised how very ill I was and told my father I must stay where I was so that I could get better. I was terrified. I was seen by nurses, doctors and social workers. The diagnosis was that I was having an acute psychotic episode. Apparently twenty five per cent of rape victims go on to develop depression and or other mental illness - which is a shocking statistic.

My work colleague told Caroline I was in hospital and she came straight there to see me that very day. I remember her visit vaguely. She says I looked even thinner, almost skeletal. I was sitting up in bed - there were curtains dividing us from the next bed, and I had my arms stretched out in front of me, with my fingers clawed. I can remember doing this. Apparently I kept looking at them as if they didn't belong to me. My hair looked as if I had not washed it for a while. I was too terrified to go to the bathroom on my own. I was quite calm – obviously drugged – but puzzled and confused as to where I was.

I knew who Caroline was and was friendly but distant. She gathered I had not had a choice in being admitted to the hospital and I was not really sure why it had happened.

For the first eleven days, I refused all food and drink. I believed myself to be dead or thought I might be in metamorphosis. Why did I need to eat and drink? My mother tried to feed me from a spoon. A friend brought me my favourite bananas to try and tempt me into eating. She said my lips were cracked and dry.

My life was perceived to be in danger and the psychiatrist told my family that I should be sectioned. He said he was saving my life rather than my sanity. The social worker did not agree with the psychiatrist. She refused to sign the forms. She told my parents she was worried I would lose my job. My parents begged her to sign the forms saying they were not worried about my job, They wanted me to be well. And so I was sectioned for twenty eight days under the 1983 Mental Health Act. Although, ironically I did start to eat and drink voluntarily almost immediately after I was sectioned, I was still catatonic and mute.

My sister Jane, who had come to visit me, was shocked when she looked into my eyes. She said they were "dead"; there was no light in them. She felt she had lost me and was dreadfully upset. I remember Jane's husband visiting me too, with their baby son in a sling, and other family and friends coming to see me.

Caroline came to the hospital to visit me again and she tells me that the nurse came out to see her before she found me. She took her into an office and told her that I had the right to challenge being sectioned and that it was important that someone I knew and trusted, explained that to me before it was too late (there was a time limit). She was concerned and quite insistent that Caroline spoke to me about it. Caroline has since told me she was very, very anti Electro Convulsive Therapy, based on the time she had spent visiting people in a mental hospital in Bristol when she had been reading for her Psychology Degree. She was already extremely unhappy about what was happening to me.

When Caroline got to me that day I was distressed, crying and terribly confused. She took time to explain to me that I did not have to just accept what was happening to me and that I could have a say in it. By then, she observed, I had lost all confidence. I didn't think I wanted to stay there but I was frightened of everyone and I didn't want to make a decision that might make anyone angry. When Caroline finished her visit that day she left the appeal forms with me and I said to her, "I think I want to sign this but I'm not sure if I can". Caroline tells me she still was not convinced I was not just under the influence of the drugs that they were keeping me sedated on.

Caroline came to see me one more time. She was living a long way away by then. She had appealed to the Mental Health Board on my behalf by fax at five minutes to midnight on the deadline day since I had not appealed myself. She had kindly found a solicitor in Kent who had agreed to put my case.

My mother was completely furious. I didn't know all the details until much later but apparently she phoned Caroline to tell her how dreadful she was.

On the day of my appeal I do remember being helped along the corridor by my mother as we walked into the room to sit before the Appeals Board. I was physically very weak and found walking difficult. I was also very drowsy from all the medication I was taking. I was terrified of the doctors on the panel and this showed.

The result of the interview was that I was too ill to be released from the section and was then sectioned again under the I983 Mental Health Act, for up to six months rather than the month I had been sectioned for initially. So my fate was sealed; I had to stay in the hospital and continue the treatment whether I wanted to or not.

The solicitor phoned Caroline to tell her the result and said that, given that she lived 150 miles away and I would be dependent on my family in Kent to support me, it was his advice that she should stay away and minimise the chances of another almighty row, with me caught in the middle. Some time afterwards I phoned Caroline apparently and said she had done the wrong thing in trying to get me out – but Caroline says it didn't sound like me. I was quite disapproving I am told, and I also said my sister Jane was mad at Caroline too. That was the last time Caroline and I spoke until I managed to trace her some years later. Thankfully we are back in touch again and our friendship has remained intact.

Other friends who visited me commented that it was difficult to tell the patients from the staff since none of the staff wore uniforms. Two work colleagues said they found me in bed when they visited and that I cheered up visibly on their arrival but when members of my family came into the room I appeared to be miserable again. My colleagues said I made it obvious I did not want to be in hospital. My mother said it was the hardest thing ever, to have to leave me there after visiting times, when she wanted to take me home with her.

Various tests were carried out on me. Some I declined to take part in, especially any where I had to lie down inside a machine. I remember one day I was taken to another part of the hospital for some tests I was very frightened of and a male nurse dragged me by my arm down the corridor.

I spent hours and hours sitting alone on my hospital bed, clutching piles of bedclothes, some of which I had taken from other patients' beds, or wandering around the unit clutching sheets. I was terrified of the other patients. And of many of the staff. Mealtimes were a frightening ordeal for me because I had to sit with other people and I was still confused about my whereabouts. Sometimes I wondered if I was on a film set. My mother wrote a moving poem about my confusion at this time and I have attached this poem "When" at the end of this book. I sometimes wondered if I had been sent on a course, other times I wondered if I was on a plane. I just did not know. I continued to hallucinate until the right mix of medication was found for me.

One day the realisation dawned; I was in hospital and my mother tried to assure me I was safe. But I felt far from safe and yearned to be home yet I knew I had no one in my house to return to. I continued to endure very frightening hallucinations and my medication was constantly changed in an attempt to   find a drug which would help me. There was a painting on the wall in the ward, of a small child sitting with a dog by her side. I was drawn to this painting, believing the girl to be me. I hallucinated that I had been abandoned in the basement of an old house and was left there alone. I also hallucinated that I had fallen down into a manhole and was trapped at the bottom of a very deep well, I kept hearing the song "ding dong bell, pussy down a well".

I would find it very confusing to see only my face in a mirror and not the rest of my body. It made me feel convinced my head was separated from my body. My head was full of odd thoughts. At the same time I would see kaleidoscopes of vivid colour swirling in front of my eyes.

None of these anti-psychotic drugs work very quickly. They can take between two weeks and a month to work. When every day in the psychiatric unit feels like a lifetime the delay can be indescribably hard to bear. It is   sometimes hard to express exactly what it feels like to experience an acute psychotic episode. I can only say that the underlying feeling is of sheer terror. I felt under constant threat and as though death was imminent at all times and always felt relieved at the end of a sequence of hallucinations that I was alive, if not alive and well.

When I came to read my medical notes I found reports that I was very variable according to which staff I was with and would veer from being quite animated to quite withdrawn.

Well-meaning people said to me I should say to myself: 'go away bad thoughts'. This was unhelpful. I realised   I had no control over how I felt or over what passed through my troubled mind. All I could do was wait for the medication to restore my brain to normal.

I know flames and fires featured a lot in my hallucinations and I have since wondered if this was a symbolic representation of all the anger I had suppressed in my life. The energy rush of the psychosis was quite incredible – almost orgasmic, but in a sinister sort of way. Some of the imagery will stay in my mind forever, of distorted bodies trapped in a huge net at the bottom of the sea, or the collapse of an oil rig; of Siamese twins and severed limbs.   There was also the feeling of travelling at speed on a fast rollercoaster, of being hurled from this rollercoaster at a fairground, of imagining I was pregnant, too. Bubbling oil and oil rigs often featured in the hallucinations and the oil rig was on the verge of collapse.

The words "eternal" and "eternally" were repeated over and over in my mind, but I heard the voice of my aunt, Audrey, and sometimes I would hear the voice and see the face of my cousin Joan who has since died. Or would see cartoon like pictures and see the words "sole survivor" or go back in my mind to Genesis and Adam and Eve or think about the Roman alphabet or have a picture in my mind of a Camel Passing

Through The Eye of A Needle. In the night I would imagine I could send mental messages to my friends Maggie or Julie or that I could hear my sister Jane's voice. I would see brightly coloured pictures in the room and have songs playing in my mind, especially those by Marvin Gaye. I would visualise extravagant Busby Berkeley musicals and sometimes the chattering of nonsense words in my mind became exhausting.

During the psychotic episode in 1993, the voices I heard in my head were sometimes female and sometimes male. The voice would usually make a running commentary on what I was doing or make a summary of what I had just done. The phrases would become repetitive. I knew the voices were manifestations of my own thoughts and learned to ignore them until they disappeared.

The visual hallucinations were something quite different and much more terrifying. While in hospital I had one where I was lying in a field which was being ploughed by a huge agricultural machine and the huge blades came sweeping across me slicing off my head. But I was an observer; it seemed to happen in front of me on a huge cinema screen.

Other hallucinations took the form of being able to see strange shapes and objects superimposed on everyday things. Any lights became terrifying and my fear of fires was heightened. I became very nervous if I saw a nurse smoking or a patient left a burning cigarette on the window sill and then walked off somewhere.

I was in a constant state of fear anyway, believing all my family to have been wiped out in a nuclear holocaust and I remember being absolutely delighted to see them when they visited me, quite unharmed, or to receive a card or letter from them. The visits of family and friends maintained some sort of reality for me and reassured me that the strange things that went on in my mind when people I knew were not there, were not going to harm me and were all part of something in my brain that would eventually settle down.

Terror followed me all through the day, at some points I was too frightened to bathe alone and had to lose my inhibitions and ask a nurse to help me, or I would be too nervous to go to the toilet on my own, I was frightened I was being observed through the mirror on the bathroom wall. Sometimes I imagined my internal organs had been cut out or I had transistors in my eyeballs. I was terrified of the microwave oven, especially when the timer counted down to zero, when I imagined there would be an explosion.

Similarly I feared an explosion when the kettle reached boiling point. Sometimes I couldn't bear to watch television in the hospital because I thought it was all about me. I also imagined that something sinister would happen on the hour every hour. I was often fearful that I would be made to dive into a swimming pool and swim underwater. If the staff ever asked me to do something I would always ask them, "What's the deadline?"

All these things were made more difficult as I was in the company of people often more ill than I was which added to my sense of persecution and fear. For weeks I was too scared to go into the psychiatrist's office and would only go to the door, or sit on the chair with him for a few seconds before leaving in a state of terror. I could not verbalise what was wrong. I was puzzling and puzzling to understand what was happening to me.

I was delighted the day my gran came to visit me. She had promised me she would. I was fighting hard to stay awake as I was so heavily medicated. I could hardly keep my eyes open. She brought me some slippers. It made my day to see her.

In all I stayed in the unit for six long months. About half way through my stay in the Victorian hospital we were all moved twenty miles to a new mental health unit near where I lived. At last I had my own bedroom. From my window I could see the buses and realised how near I was to my home. This lifted my spirits considerably even though the move itself was very unsettling for me and I relapsed a little initially. During my time in the psychiatric unit I continued to feel isolated and frightened and forgotten about.

Many of the staff did not have any understanding of what I was going through and seemed reluctant to stop and talk to me. They paid little attention to me nor to my anxieties about being there, about being separated from my loved ones and friends. Once at midnight, I was very distressed, tearful and lonely and needed to talk to someone and be reassured. The nurse on duty would not talk to me. She said I must wait until the morning because she had to give out the medication. This was the last thing I wanted to hear. I was distraught. I cried myself to sleep. My sense of rejection was overwhelming.

On another day another nurse was sitting reading a novel and when I asked to speak to her she said she couldn't as she wanted to finish her book. I could not believe what I heard. The psychiatrists seemed very remote and only seemed interested in prescribing medication and telling me that the symptoms I had were all part of the illness, yet they never named the illness or explained what the illness was.

I would like to say that the help I received from the staff was constructive or comforting but I cannot. I can only say that the sense of isolation I felt was not helpful. Resources may be stretched but when one is psychotic it is important to receive reassurance and to know staff can give their time.

One psychiatrist was very taken aback when I asked her if she had ever taken the anti-psychotic medication she had prescribed me, herself. I was upset by the many side-effects. The main one is weight gain, as the medication makes you crave carbohydrates and you feel constantly starving hungry. It is not a normal hunger, it is a desperate hunger. I would fall on food if it was brought to me by a relative or if a relative took me to the coffee bar in the hospital – it must have looked like I had not eaten for days. In fact I was so petrified of the other patients I would ask if I could go to the dining room last of all so that I could eat unaccompanied, otherwise I would not eat my meals at all, such was my fear. I would resort to selecting sandwiches which I could eat in my room. My behaviour was misinterpreted on the part of the staff as my own inability to care for myself and they said I needed prompting to eat. What they failed to understand was my fear of sitting with other patients.

Another horrid side effect was blurred vision. This really upset me as I did love to read. I had to have spectacles prematurely to counteract this problem. The blurred vision occurs because the medication plays havoc with the muscles of the eye responsible for focussing.

I also suffered from fluid retention. My ankles were very swollen and at one point I had to wear shoes two sizes bigger than my normal size. I had to be given potassium-saving, fast acting loop diuretics on one occasion. A reduction in saliva made my mouth uncomfortably dry and I would wake up with my tongue stuck to the roof of my mouth. The dentist gave me an oral spray to keep my mouth moist as he was worried about the dryness of my gums and my vulnerability to tooth decay.

My GP had to prescribe artificial tear drops to make my dry eyes feel more comfortable. Postural Hypotension was a major problem. If I got up out of bed too quickly I would feel very faint because the medication caused my blood pressure to fall. So I would have to lie flat on the bed for several minutes and then get up again. Even though I do not take medication now I still sit on the bed and count up to twenty before I stand up. It is a habit which has stayed with me.

My scalp became horribly dry and scaly and I needed a prescription to clear up the problem. I had to take the drug *Procyclidine* in conjunction with my antipsychotic medication as Parkinsonism can result so *Procyclidine* reduces the symptoms of Parkinson's disease. I am grateful to Rikki L Macdonald DipHe Mental Health Nurse, who pointed out that *Procyclidine* actually reduces the pyramidal side-effects of antipsychotic medications. The BNF *British National Formulary* (British Medical Association and the Royal Pharmaceutical Society of Great Britain) states "The antimuscarinic drugs, benzatropine, orphenadrine, procyclidine and trihexyphenidryl (benzhexol) reduce the symptoms of parkinsonism induced by antipsychotic drugs). It was also given to me as an emergency treatment when I had a reaction to an antipsychotic drug called *Risperidone* – my jaw seemed to drop and I slurred when I spoke. The psychiatrist prescribed *Procyclidine* at half hour intervals until the symptoms disappeared and I was unable to take *Risperidone* again – it had made me see pictures before my eyes like stained glass windows in a Church and they stayed there even if I closed my eyes, which was distressing.

During my time in the psychiatric unit my weight fell by two stone to eight stone twelve pounds and my periods stopped and I became very weak. It hurt me to sit on a chair because I had lost so much fat and muscle tone.

Some of the staff were utterly unhelpful. I felt misunderstood and invisible. I soon realised that the strange things I saw and heard were only happening to me and nobody else and looking back I see I was completely detached from reality.

Being so heavily medicated was one of the worst aspects of being ill. Later I said it was like trying to play a guitar wearing boxing gloves.

I was shocked to receive a letter from my employers stating that my employment was to be terminated as I had taken so much sick leave. If I could provide a psychiatrist's report they said they might be able to arrange retirement on the grounds of ill health. The deadline was very soon and my family asked my consultant to write a report which he did, just in time, and my retirement arrangements were made. My last official working day was set for 31 March 1994.

In September 1993 I welcomed the letter from the court enclosing my decree nisi and was able to apply for the decree absolute. I felt nothing but relief.

In October 1993 Jane had arranged for her son's christening. At that time I was refusing to leave the psychiatric unit and so sadly the christening went ahead without me being there and I was sad when I saw the photographs that I had missed this important occasion in my nephew's life.

There came a point where I seemed to plateau in my recovery. I just came to a halt and stayed there. My head felt full of fog and I seemed to think and move in slow motion. My psychiatrist told my parents he would have to use Electro-Convulsive Therapy (ECT) on me as nothing else was working properly. ECT involves passing an electrical current through the brain to stimulate it. My family were divided over this. I had no say in the matter at all since I was still sectioned and, though I did not want to undergo the treatment, I was resigned to it.

The psychiatrist arranged for six treatments. I was weighed prior to this and also underwent an Electroencephalogram (EEG) to find out if there were any problems with my brain. Things were normal; all that was found was a cerebral insult. In later years I asked the psychiatrist what had caused this insult. I did wonder if it had been my first husband's violence. He had once knocked me to the ground and I had hit my head on the pavement and was concussed. The psychiatrist doubted this and said it was more likely to have been caused by stress or the medication I had been taking. I understand a cerebral insult to be a kind of lesion which heals in time.

On the morning of my first treatment I was woken very early and I showered and washed my hair before being taken by a nurse to another part of the hospital. A needle was put into the back of my hand to give me a short acting anaesthetic and I was also given a muscle relaxant. I had to lie on my back on a table and the next thing I knew, I was coming round.

In the interim, electrodes had been placed on either side of my head. This is known as bilateral ECT. These electrodes delivered an electrical stimulus. The stimulus levels recommended for ECT are in excess of an individual's seizure threshold. For bilateral ECT this is between one and one and a half times the seizure threshold. The electrical stimulus is 800 milliamps and lasts between one and six seconds.

The headache I suffered afterwards was relentless and the worst I have ever experienced. To make things worse, I knew I had to undergo the treatment another five times. I had two treatments each week.

The ECT did work. I did return to reality. I resented having the treatment and it was not pleasant but I have to concede it was helpful. Of course, if the antipsychotic medication *Olanzapine (Zyprexa)* had been available to me then, I could perhaps have avoided the ECT treatment. I was to discover later that *Olanzapine* was very effective.

In January 1994 I became more and more anxious to leave the Unit and return home and my psychiatrist kept saying I could, in a week or two. The day finally came when I was released from the sectioning and allowed to leave.

DON'T MIND ME

Chapter Twelve: Homecoming

On January 25th l994 I left the Unit for the last time. I went to stay with my father and his partner for a month. I was too well to stay in hospital or to live in the so-called Halfway House but not yet well enough to live alone. This was a difficult transitional period for me. My father and his partner helped me get the house straight and helped re-decorate some of the rooms and lay new carpet. The time passed slowly and I yearned to return home.

On the day of my return, my father stayed with me a while and then left. I suddenly felt small and impotent and very frightened. The house seemed to close in on me and I rushed upstairs to bed and hid under the bedclothes.

The next morning felt very strange. Starting again was so difficult and I had become institutionalised after six months in hospital. Living alone and not having a job were the worst aspects. My mother brought my two cats home. Popsy and Vanian soon settled back in. I was very sad that my two kittens Polly and Oscar had been re-homed. I had taken on these little creatures shortly before falling ill and hardly had time to get to know them both. I hope they both went on to have happy lives.

I went to see my doctor to tell him how I was. I asked how soon I could go back to work. He said, "Oh it's very early days. Perhaps in a year's time." I had been inactive for six months while in the psychiatric unit and my doctor told me I must go walking as much as possible to build up my leg muscles. I tried to keep busy. I did some voluntary work for the local citizens' advice bureau. I received invaluable support from Maggie Gallant from the East Kent Rethink User Forum.

I remember going to my nephew's first birthday party in May, l994 and a friend saying to me "you look glam". I still felt very nervous in social situations though and was frightened I would have to explain I had had a breakdown. Despite my fears I managed to drive to Colchester to my friends' wedding that summer.

Eventually a member of the mental health team came to see me at home and things were set in motion so that I was assigned a social worker and a support worker. I later asked my support workers what their impressions of me had been at that time. One said I seemed to have been destroyed mentally by my abusive first marriage and another said I used to stop talking in the middle of a sentence. Another said I was always very 'down' and kept my thoughts and feelings to myself.

By now I had the symptoms of obsessive compulsive disorder, OCD. I exhausted myself checking that plugs were pulled out of their sockets, that taps were not dripping, that lights were not switched on and that doors were locked. It took forever to get myself out of the front door and some days I would return to the house several times before I was certain the house was secure. I would worry about the house while out and yearn to be home again. OCD was ruining my life and the worrying thoughts were very intrusive.

I was referred for CBT, Cognitive Behavioural Therapy. The waiting list was very long   At my first appointment the psychologist explained to me how CBT worked. It was a series of techniques designed to change behaviour, thoughts and beliefs. For me it was a kind of sticking plaster technique as I did not have to talk about my painful experiences but only to acknowledge they had happened.

The techniques I learned were useful and have stayed in my mind. I had to wear an elastic band loosely round my wrist so that I could "ping" it and snap myself out of any distressing or unwanted thoughts. When I woke in the morning I was advised to focus on a painting on the wall or on a clock, so that my attention was focussed on that and this would stop the spread of unwanted thoughts through my mind. Otherwise thoughts would   spread across my mind like cracks across a ceiling.

Other techniques I learned were to listen to Baroque music which was very relaxing. I went to my sessions of CBT once a fortnight for about two years and they really helped me overcome my fears, especially of cooking with gas and electricity. I could now cook meals again without any fear of explosions and could leave the house spontaneously.

I now had the confidence to go out more and to go to a Mind day centre. This was not ideal for me as the other people who went there were depressed but it was a measure of just how much

I had recovered that I was able to go there once a week. I still met a support worker twice a week too. At this stage I could only go to places by taxi and it was some time before I found the confidence to travel by bus.

In the summer of 1994 my friend Anne and I decided to go to Ireland. I had become friends with Anne in hospital and the staff had placed us in different wards as they said we were becoming too dependent on one another. After I came out of hospital I continued to see Anne and spent a lot of time with her.

I had spoken to my friend Julie in Sheffield in July 1993 just before she left to find a property in Ireland. She had found a cottage in half an acre of land with a stream running through it and had said I would always be welcome to visit but that given my breakdown, she would believe it when she saw it!

We booked our flights and some accommodation in the City of Cork for the first few days. Our journey did not get off to the best of starts as the taxi driver got lost and he was late picking us up for the airport in London. We only just made it in time.

I could not believe I was sitting on a plane waiting for it to take off. The flight was under an hour and we soon landed at Cork airport and found a taxi to take us to our hotel.

We spent a few days exploring the City and then met up with Julie and Jim there and had a meal with them before travelling to their cottage in the remote area of Inchinteskin.

We had a lovely few days at "Maggie's Cottage". The scenery was breathtakingly beautiful and the rain soft and fresh. I told Anne and Julie that my gynaecologist had recently recommended that I have a hysterectomy. They both suggested I postpone the operation, feeling it would be too much for me at that time.

The gynaecologist saw me again shortly after my return from Ireland and said he would perform a laparoscopy first. But on thinking about it I decided I wanted the hysterectomy only. I was 38 and had given up on any idea of having children. My gynaecological problems were debilitating and I felt I would be better off having the operation.

I remember Gran phoning me the night before and she wished me the "Best of British" which really touched me. She had suffered several miscarriages and a stillbirth in her time and had also had a hysterectomy when she was under forty, as my mother had.

After the operation I felt very different. I was relieved to feel better but mourned the loss of my womb and thought, why me? After all I had been through, I was now being denied the chance of having children. But I had made the choice myself. I would have to live with it.

A few weeks after my hysterectomy I learned that my great uncle Bos (Harry) had died. Bos was my Nanny's only surviving brother. I think he died of a broken heart as he lost his beloved wife some years earlier and had continued to live alone in the same house he had lived in for most of his life, a derelict place in the Elephant and Castle. When I worked in London I visited him when I could and had been to tea several times with him and my aunt, and when I left the city I kept in touch by phone. As he died only weeks after my operation I had to miss yet another funeral and was heartbroken. His surname was Wellington and I have a miniature silver Wellington boot to remember him by.

In January 1995 I had to go out one evening to attend a meeting. I didn't really want to go to it. I drove there and the meeting finished around six thirty. I remember looking at the time as I left the house and noted it was 18.42. This stuck in my mind as I thought afterwards that had I left earlier or later I would not be telling you what happened next.

I was driving home and had stopped at a junction to turn right into a main road. I looked left and right but failed to look left again and turned too early and collided with an oncoming car. My car was written off and I was knocked out. I came round to find myself in the back of an ambulance and was able to give the paramedics my father's phone number and he came to the hospital to see me while I was checked over. I had hurt my neck and had to wear a collar and had grazed my foot where it had got stuck under the pedals and was very shaken but otherwise all right. I told the doctor I was on medication and he said that was something I had to discuss with my psychiatrist. The DVLA Medical branch was informed and I now have a restricted licence and my GP is always consulted before a new one is issued.

I was advised to stay overnight at my father's house and the night passed uneventfully. The next day we retrieved the car, made an insurance claim and I had to give a statement to the police.

The case went to court. My father went and listened to the proceedings as I was not required to attend. I was fined £175 for careless driving and points were added to my licence.

As far as driving goes, I have never felt very confident behind the wheel since the crash. I did drive for a while but the confidence went away and nowadays I am happy to be a non-driver. I do feel I will never lose my driving skills and would drive if I had to.

I recovered well from the car crash and continued to see the psychiatrist monthly. I knew that as I was not sectioned I did not have to keep taking the medication. I was alarmed about the side effects but on the other hand did not want to cut down the dosage without supervision. I took most of the medication at night and once it took effect I would fall asleep suddenly. One night I feel asleep in the middle of a phone conversation with a friend, who was alarmed. She did not know what had happened to me and alerted my family. My two sisters had to come over and wake me up to check that I was all right. I had to explain to my friend later.

My psychiatrist said I could reduce the *Amitryptyline* but would have to stay on the *Olanzapine*, the antipsychotic medication, for life.

I was unhappy with this and was relieved when a new psychiatrist agreed I could cut down the *Olanzapine*. I had cut down and come off the *Amitryptyline* with no adverse effects . Originally I had been taking 450mg. The psychiatrist said this was for "protection". I started to cut down the *Olanzapine* from 20mg.

In 1995 I was terribly sad when I had to have Popsy put to sleep. In 1996 I found the courage and confidence to fly on my own to Ireland and stay with Julie again. This did me good. In 1997 I went to see my friends in Nottingham. I was aware too how much this boosted my confidence.

In 1999 my beloved Gran died. My mother had gone to visit her as usual but there was no reply when she phoned her on the way. She found Gran slumped across a chair in the kitchen. She had died from a ruptured abdominal aorta. To be on the safe side, my doctor sent me for an ultrasound but my aorta was fine and I was told to have a repeat scan when I am sixty.

I went to my Gran's funeral and grieved. Her ashes were scattered in the grounds of the church next to the school she attended when a child in Streatham and a lovely white rose now grows in the same place her ashes were scattered. I have visited this rose and have a photo of it. I also went to the road Gran lived in as a child. Though I was not sure which number she had lived at, I felt quite weird feeling run through me as I was standing looking at the houses.

I continued to see the psychiatrist and was only taking 5mg *Olanzapine,* I changed psychiatrists again and she said if I had no psychotic symptoms I could come off the drug but must stay on 5mg for twelve weeks. The last twelve weeks seemed like a lifetime and I will always remember the day in September 2000 when I stopped taking the *Olanzapine.* After I stopped taking the

Olanzapine, I felt whole again. I felt alive and alert again. I started to dream after seven years of dreamless sleep. I began to have feelings flood back into my soul. I began to take more interest in what was going on around me and in life in general. Family and friends commented on the difference in me. One friend described me as "all lit up", Jane said she had got her sister back. She had always been used to me being witty and quick on the uptake. My intellect was blunted when I was ill; it was as if the very essence of me had vanished. With hindsight she could see that as my psychosis approached I became more uptight and serious. My fine sense of humour left me; there were no quips, the speed of response slowed. Irony was lost on me; I neither used it nor appreciated it. I took everything literally and everything became very literal. She had seen me floating in and out of detachment from reality just prior to my descent into psychosis. Now, however I was back to myself again. My humour was intact, I was sharp and alert once more.

Chapter Thirteen: Ken

I began to acknowledge how lonely I was and how I wanted companionship again. I spoke to Jane and she suggested joining a dating agency. I had already started to go out more and now had the confidence to go to the pub across the road on my own.

I sent off for the dating agency application forms and spent an hour filling them in. It was pouring with rain when I went to the post box. On the way back to the house I wondered if I had wasted my time and money.

After a few days some names and addresses arrived. I discounted one person as I thought the age gap was too big, another because he was a smoker and not divorced. I was left with one phone number. I picked up the phone and started to dial. I froze. It was harder than I thought. What was I going to say about my illness, would I be rejected because of it? I abandoned the call.

The next night I made myself dial the same number. Ken answered. He said I sounded like a Tax Inspector! I was so nervous! Anyway we chatted and got on so well that over the next few days we spoke for over five hours by phone. Next we swapped photographs. We both said we did not want to spoil things and wondered if meeting each other would do this. We agreed to meet five days after the first phone call.

I went out with my support worker that day and nervously told her what was happening. As the evening approached I became very apprehensive.

Ken said he too had been anxious   as he drove to my house and found he had stopped the car right outside it.

As Ken came up the steps to the front door my stomach was somersaulting and I had a dry mouth. But we soon relaxed and when Ken left early the next morning I knew I had met a wonderful man. He told me it was love at first sight for him – for me the feeling grew more slowly but was almost instantaneous.

He moved in with me shortly afterwards and three weeks later we got engaged. When he asked me to marry him,   I did not hesitate and said yes. We went out to choose a ring. Previously I had said   I would never marry again and had   vowed never to, but meeting such a special   man changed my mind. I then knew for certain I had never been in love before and it brought home to me how much of a sham my first marriage had been.

Ken's younger daughter was only six at this time and I did not meet her straight away. She was   upset to hear that her dad was   moving away from the area to live with me and her lower lip had trembled when she was told the news. When we first met she was understandably shy. It took some time for us to get to know each other but nowadays we get along well.

My dear nephew is only eight months older than Stephanie. They are now teenagers and have become very good friends.

Chapter Fourteen: Psychosis Returns

My life was wrecked again in February 2001 when only eight weeks after meeting Ken I started to have psychotic symptoms again. I had become very tired with all the upheaval in my life and the sudden change to my routine after living on my own for so long. Ken did not know what to make of this change in me and was very frightened. For example I became very alarmed when Ken's works van came to pick him up in the mornings. I thought it signalled disaster. One night we had gone to bed and I thought I had seven seconds to get out of the house before it blew up. I jumped out of bed, ran out of the bedroom and down the stairs and out of the front door. I then realised that I was standing outside in the cold, in my dressing gown. I came to my senses, realised what I was doing and that I had not told Ken and had left him in the house, and went back inside.

I hallucinated that my uncle was having open heart surgery and that the operating theatre was right below the bedroom; I was somehow involved too in the transportation of organs for complicated transplant surgery in Canada. I also imagined my uncle and aunt were stranded on a remote island and were searching everywhere for drinking water and for precious minerals – there was an underlying feeling that I was responsible for other people's problems and that everything was my fault. I also imagined that my late friend Geoff was communicating with me through his father, from Wales.

My mother came to see me when Ken told her what my behaviour was like. I was lying in bed and I told her I could hear music playing in my head and I told her it was Diana Ross singing "Touch me in the morning". Eventually I went to see my GP after encouragement from Jane and he started me off on 5mg *Olanzapine.* I had been very difficult about admitting that I was getting unwell again. I was in denial. The over-riding fear was of being ill again and all the horrors that entailed and being able to do nothing to stop the progress of the illness. Added to this was my overwhelming fear of going into hospital again. I saw my GP on a Wednesday. As I have said, these drugs can take over two weeks to work so by the Saturday morning I was much the same. I was hallucinating about having problems with my eyes and generally feeling fearful.

I was still frightened that there had been a nuclear war and was scared of radiation. I was very anxious that I had forgotten to protect myself in some way; I thought I needed to protect my whole body – special plasticized tips for my eyelashes and special tips for my fingernails.

Ken and my mother took me to see the GP that same morning. The doctor phoned a psychiatrist who tried his best to talk to me on the phone. The line was crackling and the psychiatrist sounded foreign – I was petrified of him - he sounded like my ex-husband and I said to my GP that I was unable to speak to him .My GP understood and then arranged for me to see a psychiatrist later the same day and Ken and my mother took me to the local hospital that afternoon. We sat and waited, and waited. By this time I was really breaking down emotionally and knew I was. I was crying and crying and felt really desperate and so very frightened.

Eventually we went in to see the psychiatrist and the first thing my mother said to the doctor was that she thought I needed Electro-Convulsive Therapy again. My mother was very anxious about me and knew that Electro-Convulsive Therapy had worked for me before. I was extremely frightened and I balked at this comment. I became every more terrified. But the doctor looked at me and then at my mother and said that I didn't need ECT and asked Ken to go and buy me a bar of chocolate and let me eat it straight away, which he did. I presume this was to raise my levels of serotonin and my levels of blood sugar. The local psychiatric unit was full so a bed was found in Ashford Kent which was an hour's drive.

My heart sank as we drove there. I was hallucinating that I was about to lose a baby and that was why we were driving to hospital. I had no change of clothes and when we found the ward at the hospital I was distraught. It broke my heart when Ken and my mother left me there and I was very upset. I was in the acute ward, a four bed ward and the staff found me a new toothbrush and soap and flannel. They did their best. That night was awful. I found the separation from Ken just unbearable and was very frightened I would now lose him. I hardly slept because the fear of losing Ken was so great.

The next day Ken and my mother returned. I felt so happy to see them. I was so much more aware this time and knew where I was. I was given a test to see how my short-term memory was and that was declared to be normal. Ken and my mother came with me when I went to see a young woman called Harriet who was a psychiatrist. The first question she asked me was did I have a happy childhood. I declined to answer that question. Ken said a look of horror passed across my mother's face. It was my mother who answered for me that no, I had not had a happy childhood.

Still I encountered staff who did not have any understanding of what I was going through. One day Ken came to visit me and the nurse said he shouldn't bother visiting me because I was in a world of my own. How cruel was that! It was visits from Ken and my family which were keeping me going and giving me hope.

After a week or so in the acute ward I was transferred to the sub acute ward where I had to share a room with another patient. I have to say I was very frightened of this woman as she talked constantly throughout the night about God and The Devil and she told me she had been a resident in the Unit for eleven months. This really filled me with fear. I went on home leave and decided I did not want to return. My GP helped me to arrange my discharge and Ken went and collected my belongings. I spent the next few days at home with my mother coming to stay with me while Ken worked. I did not improve. I would have debilitating panic attacks and hyperventilate.

I would shake from head to foot and sob. I would go into a kind of trance and imagine objects were suspended from the ceiling. I would imagine everything melting around me. One day I was very upset when my mother suggested I go back into the psychiatric unit. She rang the GP who came to see me and my admission was arranged. She rang Ken when we got there and told him where I was. I felt terribly upset and disappointed to be there.

I hated being back in the unit. I would still have recurring hallucinations that I was going to die. I would curl up on the floor and wait to die. But nothing happened. It wasn't long before I began to recover and could stay at home overnight very often and then a psychiatrist realised how well I was progressing and arranged for me to transfer to the Day Unit. Now that I had Ken in my life I had an incentive to get well and return home full time.

Ken would drop me at the Day Unit at seven in the morning and pick me up at six when he finished work. I used to take my books and writing materials and sit by myself in a room for most of the day, only joining the other patients for meals. A male nurse asked me rather aggressively why I kept refusing to attend his groups. I told him I had no need to go to any of the groups. I had gone to one once - it was awful. We had to sit in a circle and talk about our thoughts. I thought, how depressing. All it did for me was to reinforce the notion that I was ill. I wanted to listen to music, to be around lively and funny people. The first thing I had asked for on being admitted to the unit was for the staff to turn on the radio so I could listen to some music; the silence just added to the depressing atmosphere in the place anyway.

After what seemed to be a lifetime I was finally discharged in May 2001 after being asked by my social worker to chair my own discharge meeting. She told me she wasn't very good at addressing meetings. I did not reply to that. I had seen enough of psychiatrists, mental health nurses and social workers. When I was twenty five I wanted to be a social worker and sent away for the application forms. On the form it said, write below your reasons for wanting to be a social worker. When faced by that question, I could not think of a single reason!

From May onwards I continued to get better in leaps and bounds. I saw the psychiatrist from time to time, was off my medication and getting on with my life.

As December approached there was much to organise for our wedding. My friend Maggie and Ken's brother and his wife were to be our witnesses and we had the ceremony booked for 11.30 a.m. on Friday 14 December. It was the first anniversary of the day I had phoned Ken. My sister co-owned a Wine Bar at the time and we had our afternoon reception there. Although it was December the weather was bright and clear and I shall remember the day always; it was truly the happiest day of my life.

In March 2002 I was deeply upset when my beloved cat Vanian became very ill with a brain lesion and had to be put to sleep. I arranged for his ashes to be scattered at the same pet crematorium in Cambridge where Popsy's ashes were scattered in 1995.

I was psychotic again in April 2003 and January 2005. Both episodes were triggered by long periods of stress. The first episode happened after we had put up with eighteen months' noise from a neighbour. Early in April 2003 Ken's father died. I was already psychotic at the funeral which took place on a Friday. I became over alert on our return and could not sleep. Ken rang Jane very late that evening and she came to see me and pleaded with me to take a *Diazepam* as I refused to take any *Olanzapine* which would be an admission that I was psychotic. Once again I was in denial and I fought hard to avoid admitting I was ill.

Jane pleaded and pleaded with me to take a *Diazepam*. She said she was going to walk the three miles back to her house. This worried me and my fears for her were heightened by my state of mind so I made a deal with her. If she took a taxi home, I would take a *Diazepam*.

The next morning I was just as ill and my father arrived. I could hear him shouting downstairs. He came up the stairs to see me in the bedroom where I was hiding under the duvet. I shouted and screamed at him to go away and slammed the bedroom door shut. He was very upset. Jane arrived and came to sit on the bed with me. I told her I did not want to go into hospital. "No way jose", she said and put her arms round me. I was distressed and tearful. Jane says I was frightened of the rats I thought were running about under the bed. I was hallucinating but finding it very hard to verbalise what was happening in my mind. I know I imagined I was disabled and was living in a specially adapted house. I also hallucinated that everything was going to liquefy and melt down. Destruction and disintegration were two main themes of my hallucinations. My voice was very child-like I do remember that, and I remember singing.

I was very distressed and was thrashing around on the bed. Jane lay down beside me and put her arms around me and tried to reassure me. My father came into the room and totally misinterpreted what he saw. He rang the doctor and said his two daughters were fighting on the bed. The doctor arrived at the house and she came straight upstairs to see me. I had seen this doctor before and did not try to resist when she injected me with 5ml of *Haloperidol* and started me on *Risperidone.* She said I would be okay and that all the psychiatric beds were full and anyway I was not ill enough to go to hospital.

In fact I had a reaction to the new medication and had to change to *Olanzapine* which soon settled me. The psychiatrist also prescribed *Diazepam* saying that I could take it as necessary. She explained that when anxiety is unchecked and changes into agitation it is then that the psychosis can start. Having the *Diazepam* with me acted as insurance and I only ever took one or two tablets. I returned to normal very quickly but I did cancel a college course, so low was my confidence.

In the June of 2003 Ken and I went on a short break to Camber Sands. I was aware I was worrying about my eyes again and said to him one day that I didn't want to walk along the beach as it was very windy and I was worried the sand would blow into my eyes.

When we returned from the holiday I had my routine eye test at the Opticians and during the test the Optician looked very concerned and said he wanted to find out the reason for the loss of vision in my eyes. He shone a very bright light into both eyes and told me I had cataracts.

The shock was enormous. He said he would write to my doctor. He told me I would need an operation on my right eye within a year or I would not be able to see at all with that eye. I was so shaken I left the Opticians without paying for the sight test – I completely forgot. I put this right when I got home.

I cried a lot that day. I remembered Maud having cataract surgery and also my gran, Marjory. I was forty seven. I was much too young to have cataracts.

The next morning I went to see my doctor and he was very reassuring. He said I must have a blood test to rule out diabetes. That came back okay. He then referred me to the hospital to see the Consultant Ophthalmologist.

When I saw the Ophthalmologist later that summer he told me my lens opacity was different from the usual cataracts he saw. He asked me if I had ever taken *Chlorpromazine.* I said yes, I had taken large quantities of this drug in 1993. He confirmed my cataracts were the result of medication. I later found out that *Amitriptyline,*

Olanzapine and possibly other drugs could have been to blame, too.

I immediately wrote to the Health Trust setting out my claim for clinical negligence. After almost two years the NHS Litigation Service settled my claim without admitting liability.

In November 2003 I went to hospital for my cataract operation. Ken took me to the ward at eight on a Friday evening. The operation was scheduled for ten o'clock that same evening. I was nervous. A group of us were sitting in the ward. I was the youngest by many years. A nurse talked to us at length about the stringent after care that would be involved after the operation and then proceeded to put anaesthetic and antibiotic drops into my right eye, at twenty minute intervals. The drops ran down the back of my throat and my face felt peculiar.

Then a male nurse came for me and I had to sit in a wheelchair and was taken to the room next door where I met the anaesthetist. He explained he would immobilise the eye with three injections. The first one, in the soft tissue under the eye, hurt enormously. The second one hurt a little less and as the injections started to work, the third was not as painful

The anaesthetist checked that my right eye was immobilised and I was wheeled through to the operating theatre where the surgeon and his team were gowned and waiting.

I had to lie down on the operating table and my head was encased in a support block. Sheets were draped over me, covering my face but a slit remained exposing my eyes.

The operation began. A small incision was made in my right eye and the clouded lens was broken down by a special process so it became emulsified and could be sucked out through a fine tube. Then an artificial lens implant was inserted in its place. All the time, I felt no pain, but felt different sensations, some pulling, some floaty and there was the constant whoosh of running water as my eye was irrigated. The operation took around twenty minutes and finally a pad and patch were placed over my eye and the block was removed from my head and I was asked to get up very carefully and sit in the wheelchair.

The surgeon said "well done" to me as I was wheeled back to see Ken. I was then given a tablet to take. This was to reduce the pressure which would have been building up in my eye during the operation. I had tea and biscuits and was given some eye drops to take home and advised to take painkillers as soon as I got home. I felt as if someone had punched me in the eye.

We got home around eleven that night and I took *paracetamol* and we went to bed. As the anaesthetic wore off the pain in my eye intensified and I wished I had taken something stronger than *paracetamol.* I felt as if something sharp was in my eye. The pain got worse before it got better and it suddenly stopped at three in the morning. The pain had made me cry. I managed some sleep and next morning I took off the pad and patch. Things were blurry to start with but my vision soon improved.

All over the weekend I had to put eye drops in the eye every two hours. The risk of infection is very high after a cataract operation and there is actually a risk of losing the eye if an infection takes hold. After the first forty-eight hours I had to continue using eye drops four times a day for a further month.

On the Monday I returned to the Ophthalmology Department and the Consultant said my eye was fine and I could be discharged into the care of my Optician. I had an appointment in six weeks' time. At this appointment I was discharged after having an eye test for new glasses and was advised to have an eye test every year.

At the time of writing, the cataract in my left eye has grown larger and I am only weeks away from my second operation. This time I will be having anaesthetic eye drops instead of injections which should reduce the post-operative pain. I will always be angry that I developed cataracts. If only I had been warned of the possibility; perhaps I could have made different choices. The Health Trust was adamant that psychiatrists could not be expected to know about the side effects of the medication they prescribed. This response made me even more angry.

The other psychotic episodes had occurred because I took on too many tasks at once and became very tired .I had misjudged the extent of my vulnerability to stress. My GP said I must learn to say "No" with resolution. I recognised the same hallucinations recurring. I have since read *Making Up The Mind, How the Brain Creates Our Mental World by Chris Frith (Blackwell)* and I contacted Professor Frith to ask about these recurrences of the same hallucination and he replied that the dopamine receptors in the brain do take a very long time to settle down.

Staying in my own surroundings definitely hastened my recovery on both occasions and a few weeks of *Olanzapine* settled me. I had to put up with all the usual side-effects and to be free of them quickly was a real incentive to get better and come off the tablets. My main concern was for my cataract which I did not want to get any larger.

I visited my GP regularly for support and he said the main thing was to get my confidence back and I would recover well, which I did. The hardest thing for me was to start taking the medication as I felt so zombie-like on it but I knew I must take it or I would not recover. The mind is really "foggy" on medication. You will have seen those overseas link-ups on the television news where there is a few seconds' delay before the foreign correspondent answers the question from the studio. That sense of delay is what I experienced when medicated. All my senses were dulled and I felt very slow, mentally. Once off the medication I was very alert and totally on-the-ball.

In January 2005 I knew I was ready to adopt another cat and we found a young tabby called Smudge at the local rescue centre. He had been living there for seven months and had arrived there quite traumatised. He settled with us very well though and is a delight.

In late 2005 I noticed my ankles were swelling every day. I had some blood tests and it was found that in the tests for the liver the ALT (Alanine Transaminase, a transaminase enzyme) level was too high, indicating liver damage. My doctor explained that my liver was now fragile from the years of having to process all the medication. I had the test repeated after a month during which I drank no alcohol and the reading had fallen by 20 and was almost normal. I have not drunk alcohol since.

Chapter Fifteen: Reflections

Since the events of l993 my life has got better and better. In the beginning progress was very slow despite the fact that I tried very hard. I now realise that the mind and body take an extraordinarily long time to recover from the shock of psychosis. I found the process of starting again akin to trying to complete a jigsaw puzzle without a picture to work with. I found that patience was the key to recovery. In the early days there were times when my anxiety was so high that I could not move out of the kitchen all day; I was terrified to walk down our own stairs into the basement or up our own stairs to the bedroom. I would have to divide up the day into hours and get through each hour, little by little. I wrote down what I was doing and used a notebook to note each hour that passed. Motivation had left me. I sorely missed the structure a job gives to the week. I missed seeing colleagues. I missed having anything meaningful to do. I was constantly warned not to stress myself. I felt like a prisoner. I would make a list of things to do. I would make myself walk to the post box and post a letter. My pace would quicken as I reached the house and once indoors again I would relax. The ordeal was over. Then I would walk further, to the shops.

Nature took its course and my brain settled. I tried to do more and more each day and increase my motivation and confidence. Past stresses had accumulated and added to the grieving process from the loss of loved ones, building up until something had to give. I always liken it to a saucepan coming to the boil and then boiling over. Now my tortured mind needed time to heal itself.

Eventually I found enough confidence to sign up for a computer course at college. My spirits lifted, I signed up for a twelve week course in music and movement. I started an Open University course in social sciences but lacked the confidence to go away to the residential summer school so had to cancel.

I went to a daytime yoga class and then found the confidence to go to the gym under the supervision of a trainer and gradually built up my strength.

I started an A level course in Sociology but found it difficult to go to evening classes by myself and lost interest in the course. I went to a daytime pottery class which I enjoyed immensely and did some daytime voluntary office work.

As my confidence has increased I have been able to study proof-reading at home . I went to college for two half day seminars, in Autism Awareness and Dyslexia Awareness. The latter was especially helpful to me as my husband Ken is dyslexic and I had spent a lot of time researching the condition. I first contacted the Dyslexia Research Trust, based at The University of Oxford and their support was invaluable. Through the DRT I learned about FAB Research http://www.fabresearch.org , a charity examining the link between food and behaviour set up by Dr Alex Richardson who led the Durham Fish Oils Trials. I am a voluntary newshound for FAB - something I really enjoy. I became an associate member of FAB and have now been made an honorary life associate member in recognition of my continuing contribution.

I have been at college studying the Maths I was forced to drop at school and passed the GCSE exams in the summer of 2008. I am now studying science.

I have joined the University of the Third Age and completed two online courses. I take a great interest in current   affairs.   I love football and have supported Chelsea FC for over four decades.   I enjoy going fishing with Ken and riding pillion on his motorbike.

My life now is very different but my quality of life is excellent and I feel useful. I have lost my initial embarrassment about being ill and having to explain why I retired from work at thirty nine. One in four people has a mental illness and it can happen to absolutely anybody. We are all as vulnerable as each other. I have thought about my life and wondered how I fit into the ongoing Nature v Nurture debate. It is now becoming clear that a foetus is affected by the stress its mother experiences and this stress can raise the levels of cortisol, the stress hormone in the unborn child and such stress can be measured in the foetus and indeed lead to psychosis in later life "*Recently, an even wider range of adult-related chronic disorders, including osteoporosis, mood disorders and psychoses, have been intimately linked to pre- and perinatal developmental influences'. (Gluckman and Hanson 2004) The Biology of Belief by Bruce Lipton PhD (Cygnus Books) The Biology of Belief* presents the scientific evidence showing that our genes and DNA do not control our biology. Rather, genes are turned on and off by signals from outside the cell, including the energetic messages coming from our positive and negative thoughts. '*Epigenetics, the study of the molecular mechanisms by which environment controls gene activity, is today one of the most active areas of scientific research*' Dawson Church's *The Genie in Your Genes (Cygnus Books)* outlines the new scientific research showing that many genes are changing constantly through our beliefs our thoughts and our attitudes. Previously the idea was that we inherited our genes from our parents and these could make us susceptible to mental illness. As I have said there are depressive genes in my family gene pool but having read *The Genie in Your Genes* and *The Biology of Belief* I believe it has been my upbringing and general environmental influences that have led to my susceptibility to psychosis. I think we can underestimate just how much the unborn baby, the young baby, toddler and child can and does absorb through observing his parents and how their actions can shape the child's life, beliefs and thoughts, *The Healing Power of EFT and Energy Psychology* by David Feinstein, Donna Eden and Gary Craig, (*Piatkus*) shows how we can tap into the body's energy to change our lives. Gary Craig developed *Freedom Technique EFT* which taps on specific points on the skin to send electrochemical signals directly to the brain (www.emofree.com).

When I compare and contrast my own life with that of my sister, I can see that whereas my own development in my mother's womb was very stressful my sister was conceived in an atmosphere of relative calm and my mother's second pregnancy was a much happier time. My sister rarely cried and was a very calm and contented baby. I was a very tearful baby. After all, my mother lived through much stress and unhappiness while carrying me and I absorbed much of this. My sister has never been psychotic.

Having a mental illness certainly showed me who my true friends are. There are friends who have stood by me and remained in touch with me, constantly offering support and encouragement. They lost me as a friend for a while but they got me back again and our friendship is stronger because of what happened. Some friends have been unable to understand me and have drifted away.

My sister Jane Wenham-Jones has written about mental illness and in her first novel *Raising The Roof* (Bantam Books) the character Juliette is based on me. Jane asked me if she could base a character on me and I said no, I didn't mind, and then waited for her to ask me for first-hand information but instead she asked others to describe my admission to the psychiatric unit. Jane has later explained that she really wanted to have an observer's viewpoint and at that time, my recollections were blurry.

When Jane first gave me a copy of *Raising The Roof* I was very upset. I felt parodied! I then realised Jane had written about me with deep love and understanding and that it had been very therapeutic for her to write about my illness, through the characterisation of Juliette.

I quote:

'I don't know what I felt when I looked at her then. Some huge sense of loss and displacement, guilt at my rising sense of horror and recoil. This person sitting in front of me was not my sister Juliette. It was not her but I could see the place where she used to be.
Her eyes widened again and filled with tears. "I'm afraid," she said breathlessly. Her tongue dabbed anxiously at her dry, cracked lips.
"I think," the words came in short bursts, "when you get in the car," her voice was high and trembling, "it will explode and you'll die"
"Don't be ridiculous," I snapped, alarmed, "Nothing whatsoever will happen to me."
She was crying again'.

   But when psychosis takes over the brain, it cannot differentiate between normal things and things that are dangerous, so danger is seen in every situation and when one's fears are disregarded by others it is very difficult to understand why other people are not as fearful as you are. What you are looking for at this time is collusion really and support too.
   I take the next quotes from Jane's article *The Dark Side* (The Guardian, August 6, 2005)

'"If one in four of us suffer from depression, then three-quarters of the population have a hell of a lot

to put up with. It is a sad fact that we are more sympathetic to physical disease, but it is not hard to see why. Once, sitting in the bleak mental-health unit of the local hospital, I got talking to a woman whose partner was having a 12th session of ECT in the hope of being jolted out of a deep, debilitating despair. Comforting me in my guilt and helplessness over my own relative, she said. "Just give what you have to give, because you could throw your whole life in there. Depression is a black hole. It will swallow you up and still never be enough." '

I do feel for my sister, but unless you have experienced the dragging greyness of depression or the suffocating terror of psychosis you will never be able to understand just what it is like and how helpless and impotent it makes you feel. You struggle to claw your way out but until your brain settles all your efforts are futile.

In 2006 I decided I no longer wanted to be under the supervision of the local mental health team. It was a stigma I could do without. I had not used their services since 2003 and rarely saw a psychiatrist. I had to attend a meeting with a psychiatrist I had never met, and a social worker I had met once. I was adamant I wanted to leave and be placed under the care of my GP. I repeated my request over and over. Amazingly the social worker said she had not realised the element of stigma involved in being kept on the books of the team and not using their services. After the psychiatrist talked to my GP, the arrangements were put in place and I finally received a letter saying I had been discharged.

In 2007 I decided I needed to write an account of my illness. This was cathartic for me. I wrote an article and it was published in *Mental Health Practice* magazine in June 2007. A photographer came and took some photos of me on the beach looking very thoughtful and one of these appeared with the article. I was then encouraged by Jason Pegler at *Chipmunkapublishing* to write this book about my life, my illnesses and my recovery. I had found my voice.

Being married and a stepmother makes me feel valued. I still have mixed emotions about my hysterectomy. The feelings of loss stay with me. Step motherhood has been the steepest learning curve of my life. Building a relationship with a stepchild takes time and sensitivity; it is a real balancing act for all concerned. Ken and I are still very much in love and are the best of friends.

Nowadays I am still living my life free of medication and my GP is happy for things to stay that way, provided I take the medication if and when it becomes necessary. I don't feel I want to take medication as protection and feel that to take medication when I am well is like taking an aspirin in case I get a headache. As time goes by the risk of a relapse lessens but of course it will always be there.

Having a difficult and painful childhood has made it hard for me to relate well to my parents. It is only recently that my mother and I have really got on with each other. It was very hard for me to forget the past. Writing about it has helped me to forget. My father has mellowed slightly as he has aged. Above all, I value myself and believe in myself now, and that has been a major step forward. I try to sleep well and eat well and take fish oils, which contain EPA and promote mental acuity. Music has always been important in my life and so has reading and writing. And where would I be without my sense of humour! I lost my sense of humour when I was ill and felt as if a part of me was missing. When it returned I felt complete. I have worked hard on myself. I know myself better now.   I have   endured much ignorance about mental illness. I even heard the psychiatric unit called the Nut House.   One friend found me difficult to be with after my first psychotic episode and told me I had lost my "sparkle". Another friend who had never experienced depression was impatient with me when I finally told her about my mental breakdown, saying "Life's too short for nervous breakdowns"' I say, try to be patient with somebody who has a mental illness, they cannot help it, they did not ask for it to happen.

I suffered a devastating mental illness which changed the course of my life; it terrified me; it crept up on me, silently and like a thief it snatched away my mind and my dignity for a time. And yes, as each day passes I offer thanks for the fact that I am well. The fear of being ill again is always there but I am growing stronger and stronger every day. The illness in I993 was the most debilitating event in my life so far. I suppose I had to lose my mind to find it again.

DON'T MIND ME

Afterword

In 1994, my mother wrote a long narrative poem
about my descent into psychosis, and recovery
through ECT. We had frequent discussions as the
poem was being written with my mother's
observations   and all the powerful imagery
that came to me out of my experience.
   Now she has reworked the structure of that
 poem especially for *Don't Mind Me,* while
keeping all my original imagery connecting to
my feelings and perceptions during
my hospitalization.

A poem for Judith

When

I'm on a film set in a studio.
I hear the other actors say
words   without meaning. Words come and go
around me . I play the part
of silent outsider. There is no
director or direction, yet voices are clear,
repeating words I do not want to hear,
or speak. My mouth is dry. I shake my head, 'No'
to the tired woman who asks me
if there's something I want to say.
Filming goes on all day.

I'm playing guitar with boxing gloves
knocking myself down like dead wood
and marking more distance
between me and whoever else I am.

My mother is called in on the set.
She's word-perfect today, and I let
her kiss me. She says she loves me.
She's really professional with the crying.
I want to tell her she's good,
but the bloody gloves and mouth shield
dumb me down. The voices say she's lying.

I don't want her to go
when filming is over for the night
when she's fed me spoon by slow spoon
when I'm fighting to stay awake
when I've stood in line for medication,
when she's waving from the door -
when the door is unlocked the next morning
when I've unwound myself from foetal coil
when someone wakes me to start filming
when the voices tell me what to do
when I'm playing guitar with boxing gloves
when someone takes me somewhere different -

I wake up. I am safe.No voices deny it.
My mouth is fluid present tense.
I interrupt my mother asking me how I feel -
I feel alive!
My ungloved hands feel alive.
I could pick up my guitar.

Resources

The following sources of help and advice have been useful to me and I would like to share them with you.

Stand to Reason is a service led organisation working with and for people with mental ill health. ***Stand to Reason*** intends to work in a similar way to that in which Stonewall has for gay people; raising the profile, fighting prejudice, establishing rights and achieving equality.
http://www.standtoreason.org.uk

Living Life To The Full is a powerful free online life skills resource. This course has been written by a psychiatrist who has many years experience using a Cognitive Behavioural Therapy (CBT) approach. http://www.livinglifetothefull.com

Database of Individual Patient Experiences (***DIPEx***)
DIPEx offers a wide range of personal experiences of health and illness
http://www.dipex.org

SPN Social Perspectives Network

A unique coalition of service users, survivors, carers, policy makers, academics, students and practitioners interested in how social factors both contribute to people becoming distressed and play a crucial part in promoting people's recovery
http://www.spn.org.uk

SANE offers information and support and carries out research into mental illness
http://www.sane.org.uk

Mind - leading mental health charity in England and Wales working for a better life for everyone experiencing mental distress
http://www.mind.org.uk

Rethink - leading national mental health charity working to help everyone affected by severe mental illness recover a better quality of life
http://www.rethink.org

Your Voice in Sheffield Mental Health, a magazine for users, carers and professionals
http://www.yourvoicesheffield.org.uk

Birmingham City University CCMH Centre for Community Mental Health works to improve services and life opportunities for people with severe and enduring mental health problems
http://www.ccmh.uce.ac.uk

The National Service User Network serves to develop links and networking in order to engage and support the widest range of mental health service users and survivors across England. http://www.nsun.org.uk

One In Four is an innovative and inspirational magazine aimed at anyone
with   mental health difficulties. The features are mainly written by those with
mental   health difficulties themselves.
http://www.oneinfourmag.org

Heal Your Mind: a website covering a range of views about mental health
Whether pro or anti psychiatry.
http://www.healyourmind.org.uk

Shift. An initiative to fight the stigma and discrimination surrounding mental
health issues in England.   http://www.shift.org.uk

 Madness Explained – Psychosis and Human Nature
Richard P Bentall (Penguin)

NET.mesomoco.org.uk   Gated to ensure privacy, this social network is exclusively for the mental health community.
http://www.NET.mesomoco.org.uk.

Mental Health Today Magazine
http://www.mentalhealthtoday.co.uk

Mental Health Practice Magazine
http://www,mentalhealthpractice.rcnpublishing.co.uk

Professor DL Edmunds Ed.D, Leader of the world wide humane psychiatry movement
http://www.DrDanEdmunds.com

The Patients Voice: a forum where patients, their families and friends can participate in a wide variety of market research projects about health care and medicine
http://www.thepatientsvoice.org The Patients Voice *icarecafe* is a global network for patients and their families http://www.icarecafe.com

References

Chapter Ten: Alone –My Descent Into Psychosis

Beyond Fear by Dorothy Rowe (Harper Collins)
www.dorothyrowe.com.au

Chapter Eleven – Hospital

*British National Formulary (*British Medical Association, Royal Pharmaceutical Society of Great Britain. http://www.BNF.org

Chapter Fourteen – Psychosis Returns

Making Up The Mind by Chris Frith (Blackwell Pulbishing)

Chapter Fifteen – Reflections

Raising The Roof by Jane Wenham-Jones (Bantam Books)
http://www.janewenham-jones.com

FAB Research http://www.research.org

The Biology of Belief, Unleashing the Power of Consciousness, Matter and Miracles by Bruce Lipton PhD (Cygnus Books)
http://www.brucelipton.com

The Genie In Your Genes, Epigenetic Medicine and the New Biology of Intention
By Dawson Church (Cygnus Books)
http://www.EpigeneticMedicine.org

The Healing Power of EFT and Energy Psychology by David Feinstein, Donna Eden & Gary Craig (Piatkus)
http://www.EnergyPsychEd.com
http://www.EnergyMed.info
http://www.emofree.com

The Dark Side by Jane Wenham-Jones (*The Guardian* August 6, 2005)
http://www.guardian.co.uk

My Mental Health by Judith Haire, *Mental Health Practice* June 2007
http://www.mentalhealthpractice.rcnpublishing.co.uk

'When' Anon 2008

Printed in the United Kingdom
by Lightning Source UK Ltd.
134094UK00001B/73-90/P